PERTUSSIS - DISEASE, CONTROL AND CHALLENGES

Edited by **Waldely Dias** and **Isaias Raw**

Pertussis - Disease, Control and Challenges
http://dx.doi.org/10.5772/intechopen.70021
Edited by Waldely Dias and Isaias Raw

Contributors

Salvatore De-Simone, Giovanni Gabutti, Armando Stefanati, Parvanè Kuhdari, Daniela Hozbor, Filumena Maria Da Silva Gomes, Maria Helena Valente, Ana Maria Escobar, Sandra Josefina Ferraz Ellero Grisi, Waldely Dias

Notice

First published in London, United Kingdom, 2018 by IntechOpen
IntechOpen is the global imprint of INTECHOPEN LIMITED, registered in England and Wales, registration number: 11086078, The Shard, 25th floor, 32 London Bridge Street
London, SE19SG – United Kingdom
Printed in Croatia

British Library Cataloguing-in-Publication Data
A catalogue record for this book is available from the British Library

Additional hard copies can be obtained from orders@intechopen.com

Pertussis - Disease, Control and Challenges, Edited by Waldely Dias and Isaias Raw
p. cm.
Print ISBN 978-1-78923-528-9
Online ISBN 978-1-78923-529-6

For EU product safety concerns:
IN TECH d.o.o., Prolaz Marije Krucifikse Kozulić 3, 51000 Rijeka, Croatia,
info@intechopen.com or visit our website at intechopen.com.

Meet the editors

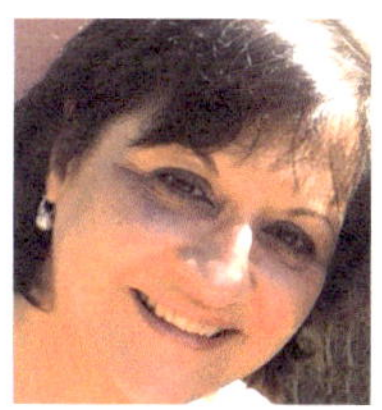

Dr. Waldely Dias graduated in Biomedical Sciences at the Federal University of São Paulo (1977) and obtained her Master's degree (1981) and PhD (1983) in Microbiology and Immunology at the same university. She has completed post-doctoral fellowship at the Institut Pasteur Paris, in the Laboratory of Biotechnologies - Hybridolab (1987) and at the Food and Drug Administration (FDA) - Laboratory of Pertussis, USA (1992). As a senior scientific researcher of the Biotechnology Center at the Butantan Institute (now Special Laboratory of Vaccine Development) since 1988, Dr Dias is involved in the development of new bacterial vaccines, including a whole cell pneumococcal vaccine and new alternatives for pertussis vaccines.

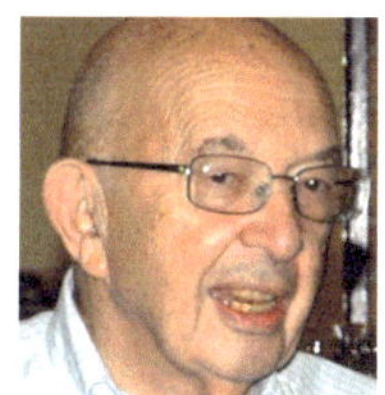

Dr. Isaias Raw graduated in Medicine at the São Paulo University (1950), having been professor of Physiological Chemistry at the Faculty of Medicine of the same University. Previous Director of Butantan Institut (1991-1997) and President of the Butantan Foundation (1998 – 2009). He founded the Biotechnology Center of the Butantan Institute, where he was director for 19 years (1983 – 2002). He has been dedicated for more than thirty years to the development of vaccines and pharmaceutical products by Butantan Institution, in production processes that result in products to be made available to the Ministry of Health of Brazil, for free use to the population.

Contents

Preface

This book aims to present an overview of the pertussis infection, focusing important issues about the diagnosis, the treatment of the disease, and the epidemiological and clinical aspects in populations with high-vaccination rates.

Current proposals for vaccination against pertussis, as well as current strategies of immunization programs, which primarily try to protect susceptible young children in the first year of life, who have not yet been immunized or are with incomplete vaccination schedule, will also be addressed.

Despite the effective and safe alternatives for immunoprevention, several challenges still have to be overcome for control of the disease, which remains a highly relevant problem in public health in terms of morbidity and mortality, with an increasing incidence even in countries with high-vaccine coverage.

We would like to thank all those who contributed to the realization of this work, especially the authors, for the content of the chapters of high-scientific value. We would also like to thank InTechOpen publishing team and Ms. Marijana Francetic for the technical support.

Waldely Dias and Isaias Raw
Instituto Butantan
Center of Biotechnology
Special Laboratory of Vaccine Development
São Paulo, Brazil

Section 1

Introduction

Chapter 1

Introductory Chapter: Pertussis - Disease, Control and Challenges

Waldely Dias

Additional information is available at the end of the chapter

http://dx.doi.org/10.5772/intechopen.77134

1. Introduction

Since that the smallpox vaccine became available in the late eighteenth century, a significant number of diseases were gradually being controlled by vaccines, which are currently considered the most successful and cost-effective intervention in public health [1]. Recent data from Gavi - the Vaccine Alliance [2] in a survey for 10 immunopreventable diseases in 41 developing countries, indicate vaccines will prevent 36 million deaths between 2016 and 2030. The impact of vaccination extends from "saving lives" to socioeconomic aspects, in a line of cause and effect between health and social productivity. After almost 70 years, vaccination around the world ended up exerting selective pressure in the microbial environment, so it is now virtually impossible to know how it would be like if the vaccines had not been introduced.

However, the control of microorganisms by the vaccines may lead the population to the false impression that pathogens responsible for devastating epidemics in the past centuries are definitively extinguished. As a consequence, the refusal of vaccines, for religious or philosophical questions, or even for discredit on the effectiveness and safety of these products is becoming a growing concern. This change in population behavior, fueled by the relatively recent technology allowing for almost instantaneous dissemination of information, whether true or false, has been observed in several countries, with a consequent increase in the number of cases and deaths related to infections that can be controlled by vaccines, as has been happening in relation to measles and whooping cough, in a very worrying way.

In this book, we propose some approaches about interrelationships between vaccine strategies and microbial epidemiology, taking as reference the whooping cough, an endemic disease with significant morbidity and mortality and of indisputable importance in public health.

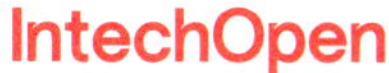

The major causative agent of pertussis, *Bordetella pertussis*, was first isolated in 1906 by Bordet and Gengou [3], and throughout that century, endemic and epidemic episodes of the disease were recorded [4].

In 1933, a vaccine which conferred a certain degree of protection was described, a suspension of killed *B. pertussis* cells [5]. In that decade and in the next, several whole cell pertussis preparations have been described and used in both prevention and treatment of the disease, with some efficacy [6]. In 1947, the Kendrick protection test was described, with intracerebral challenge in mice that is until now recommended by the WHO as an assay of potency of whole cell pertussis vaccines and the only one that showed correlation with protection in children [7]. Immunization against pertussis is part of the childhood immunization schedule and in some countries it is also recommended in booster doses for adolescents and adults [8]. Whole cell pertussis vaccines (wP), composed of inactivated suspensions of partially detoxified *B. pertussis*, have been used in vaccination programs for 60 years with proven efficacy, combined with tetanus and diphtheria toxoids adsorbed on aluminum salts as adjuvants [9]. The introduction of these vaccines in the 1950s–1960s led to a dramatic reduction of more than 90% in the incidence and mortality caused by the disease in the industrialized world [10].

Adverse reactions related to them led to development of acellular pertussis vaccines (aP), containing purified antigenic components of *B. pertussis*. These preparations are effective and less reactogenic [11], and they have replaced the (wP) in several countries in the last two decades. However, their cost of production is much higher, making prohibitive their introduction in developing countries. Preliminary clinical trials in the 1990s comparing bacterial triple vaccines formulated with diphtheria (D) and tetanus (T) toxoids combined with whole cell pertussis component (DTwP) or acellular pertussis component (DTaP), suggested similar efficacy and immunogenicity [12–16]. More recent data showed that pertussis is not adequately controlled, and epidemic outbreaks are occurring even in countries with high vaccination coverage, making the resurgence of the disease a worldwide problem [17–19].

This increase in the incidence is certainly related to multiple factors. The improved diagnostic testing, which would lead to an increase in reported cases; the decrease in vaccine efficacy and faster loss of immunity could certainly contribute to this scenario [20].

Besides that, the introduction of the aP vaccines which appear to require earlier and more frequent booster doses for disease control, suggest a shorter period of effective immunity [21]. A recent study in a systematic review and meta-analysis of published studies comparing the efficacy of wP and aP within 3 years after the 3-dose primary series concluded that the protection against the disease was lower for aP vaccines than for the wP, with efficacy of 84% and 94%, respectively [22]. The study, comparing the duration of immunity conferred by childhood vaccination scheme using 3–5 doses of DTaP, suggested that for each year after the last dose of DTaP, the disease probability would be increased 1.33 times. Assuming 85% of vaccine efficacy it was estimated that only 10% of the vaccinated children had persistence of pertussis immunity for a period of 8.5 years after the last dose [22].

Broadly speaking, aP vaccines are considered safer, but there is a currently consensus that they also require more frequent booster doses, given that they confer protective immunity for a shorter period than that elicited by wP, besides not preventing colonization and transmission after challenge [23]. Recent WHO reports confirm that wP and aP are equivalent in disease prevention in the first year of life, but that there is in fact a more rapid loss of immunity conferred by aPs [24].

In this sense, alternative pertussis vaccines have been suggested, including a live attenuated pertussis vaccine [25] and a whole cell pertussis vaccine with reduced content of endotoxin [26]. Although with efficient and safe alternatives for prevention, pertussis is still the most frequent and lethal immunopreventable disease. New vaccine options, combined with strategic actions in immunization programs, are still essential for disease control and the spread of the microorganism in the target populations.

The following chapters will focus on different aspects of the pertussis host-pathogen interrelationship. Important epidemiological aspects that may contribute to the diagnosis of the microorganism and treatment of the disease will be addressed. Current vaccine proposals, the current disease control situation and future challenges will be discussed. In this sense, it will be approached the modern vaccination strategies that aim to focus children under one year of age, mainly on the group up to 6 months, still with incomplete vaccination schedule, acquiring the infection from adults and adolescents of their conviviality. Vaccination of the mother during pregnancy a strategy that has been successfully adopted for the protection of the newborn; the currently used vaccines and the influence of high vaccination coverage strategies in the incidence of the disease should be also discussed.

Acknowledgements

We would like to thank all those who contributed to the realization of this book, especially the authors, for the content of the chapters of high scientific value. To Intechopen, for the invitation to carry out this work and to Ms. Marijana Francetic, for the technical support.

Fundings

This work was funded by the Brazilian National Bank for Economic and Social Development (BNDES), National Council for Scientific and Technological Development (CNPq) and Butantan Foundation.

Author details

Waldely Dias

Address all correspondence to: waldely.dias@butantan.gov.br

Special Laboratory of Vaccine Development, Butantan Institute, São Paulo, Brazil

References

[1] https://www.cdc.gov/mmwr/preview/mmwrhtml/mm5518a4.htm

[2] https://www.gavi.org/library/news/press-releases/2018/study-vaccines-prevent-not-just-disease-but-also-poverty/

[3] Bordet J, Gengou U. Le microbe de la coqueluche. Annales De l'Institut Pasteur. 1906;**20**: 48-68

[4] Historical review of pertussis and the classical vaccine. The Journal of Infectious Diseases. 1996;**174**(Suppl 3):8259-8263

[5] Madsen T. Vaccination against whooping cough. Journal of the American Medical Association. 1933;**101**:187-188

[6] Lapin JH. Whooping Cough. Springfield, IL: CC Thomas; 1943

[7] Xing D, Markey K, Gaines Das R, Feavers I. Whole-cell pertussis vaccine potency assays: The Kendrick test and alternative assays. Expert Review of Vaccines. 2014;**13**(10): 1175-1182

[8] WHO Expert Committee on Biological Standardization Sixty-Second Report – WHO Technical Report Series No. 979. 2011

[9] Cherry JD, Brunell PA, Golden GS, Darzon DT. Report of the task force on pertussis and pertussis immunization – 1988. Pediatrics. 1988;**81**(suppl):939-984

[10] http://www.who.int/biologicals/vaccines/pertussis/en/

[11] Zhang L, Prietsch SO, Axelsson I, Halperin SA. Acellular vaccines for preventing whooping cough in children. Cochrane Database of Systematic Reviews. 2011;**1**:CD001478

[12] Lugauer S, Heininger U, Cherry JD, Stehr K. Long-term clinical effectiveness of an acellular pertussis component vaccine and a whole cell pertussis component vaccine. European Journal of Pediatrics. 2002;**161**:142-146. DOI: 10.1007/s00431-001-0893-5

[13] Salmaso S, Mastrantonio P, Tozzi AE, Stefanelli P, Anemona A, Ciofi degli Atti ML, Giammanco A, Group SIW. Sustained efficacy during the first 6 years of life of 3-component acellular pertussis vaccines administered in infancy: The Italian experience. Pediatrics. 2001;**108**:E81. DOI: 10.1542/peds.108.5.e81

[14] Taranger J, Trollfors B, Lagergård T, Lind L, Sundh V, Zackrisson G, Bryla DA, Robbins JB. Unchanged efficacy of a pertussis toxoid vaccine throughout the two years after the third vaccination of infants. Pediatric Infectious Disease Journal. 1997;**16**(2):180-184. DOI: 10.1097/00006454-199702000-00003

[15] Edwards KM, Decker MD. Pertussis vaccines. In: Plotkin SA, Orenstein WA, Offit PA, editors. Vaccines. 6th ed. Edinburgh, Scotland: Elsevier Saunders; 2013. pp. 447-492

[16] Plotkin SA, Cadoz M. The acellular pertussis vaccine trials: An interpretation. Pediatric Infectious Disease Journal. 1997;**16**:508-517. DOI: 10.1097/00006454-199705000-00011

[17] Cherry JD. Epidemic pertussis in 2012 – The resurgence of a vaccine preventable disease. New England Journal of Medicine. 2012;**367**:785-787. DOI: 10.1056/NEJMp1209051

[18] Chiappini E, Stival A, Galli L, de Martino M. Pertussis re-emergence in the post-vaccination era. BMC Infectious Diseases. 2013;**13**:151. DOI: 10.1186/1471-2334-13-151

[19] Clark TA, Messionier NE, Hadler SC. Pertussis control: Time for something new? Trends in Microbiology. 2012;**20**:211-213. DOI: 10.1016/j.tim.2012.03.003

[20] Cherry JD. Pertussis: Challenges today and for the future. PLoS Pathogens. 2013;**9**(7): e1003418. DOI: 10.1371/journal.ppat.1003418

[21] Witt MA, Katz PH, Witt DJ. Unexpectedly limited durability of immunity following acellular pertussis vaccination in preadolescents in a North American outbreak. Clinical Infectious Diseases. 2012;**54**:1730-1735

[22] McGirr A, Fisman DN. Duration of pertussis immunity after DTaP immunization: A meta-analysis. Pediatrics 2015;**135**:331-3343

[23] Warfel JM, Zimmerman LI, Merkel, TJ. Acellular pertussis vaccine protect against disease but fail to prevent infection and transmission in a nonhuman primate model. In: Proceedings of the National Academy of Sciences of the United States of America. 2014;**111**:787-92

[24] WHO report Pertussis vaccines: WHO position paper, August 2015—Recommendations. Vaccine 34. 2016:1423-1425

[25] Locht C, Papin JF, Lecher S, Debrie A-S, Thalen M, Solovay K, Rubin K, Mielcarek N. Live Attenuated Pertussis Vaccine BPZE1 Protects Baboons Against *Bordetella pertussis* Disease and Infection, The Journal of Infectious Diseases, 1 July 2017;216(1):117-124. https://doi.org/10.1093/infdis/jix254

[26] Dias WO, van der Ark AAJ, Sakaushi MA, Kubrusly FS, Prestes AFRO, Borges MM, Furuyama N, Horton DSPQ, Quintilio W, Antoniazi M, Kyipers B, van der Zeijst BAM, Raw I. A whole cell pertussis with reduced content of endotoxin. Human vaccines and Immunotherapeutics. 2013;**9**(2):339-348

Section 2

Pertussis - Epidemiology, Diagnosis, Treatment and Immune Response

Chapter 2

Update on Epidemiology, Diagnosis, and Treatment of Pertussis

Daniela Hozbor

Additional information is available at the end of the chapter

http://dx.doi.org/10.5772/intechopen.72847

Abstract

Pertussis, commonly known as whooping cough, is one of the most common vaccine-preventable infections. In adolescents and adults, infection may result in a protracted cough and is occasionally associated with substantial morbidity. In children and particularly infants, morbidity is more often substantial and the disease may be fatal. Two types of vaccines against pertussis exist: whole-cell vaccines (wP), developed in the 1940s, containing the entire inactivated *Bordetella pertussis* organism, and acellular vaccines (aP) constituting of 1–5 purified bacterial proteins. The aPs were developed in the 1970s in order to diminish the adverse effects that could occur in the wP vaccinations. In many industrialized countries, aP replaced the wP formulations; however, wPs are still used for primary vaccination doses in developing countries. The massive use of both types of vaccines significantly reduced the morbidity and mortality associated with the disease; nevertheless, pertussis is still an important public health problem. In fact, pertussis incidence has increased in many countries, with large sustained epidemics occurring most notably in developed countries that only use acellular vaccine for all the doses included in the calendar. This chapter focuses on some recent developments in the areas of epidemiology, diagnosis, and treatment of pertussis.

Keywords: pertussis diagnosis, epidemiology, treatment

1. Introduction

Whooping cough or pertussis is a respiratory disease that though preventable by vaccination remains an important health problem not only for infants but also for adolescents and adults [1, 2]. By definition, the etiologic agent responsible for this disease is the Gram-negative bacterium named *Bordetella pertussis*. However, pertussis-like symptoms can be caused by several other *Bordetella* species, including *B. parapertussis*, *B. bronchiseptica*, and *B. holmesii* [3–8]. The

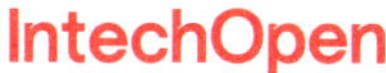

disease usually starts with cold-like symptoms and irritating cough that gradually becomes paroxysmal. Paroxysms are characterized by repeated violent coughs; each series of paroxysm has many coughs without intervening inhalation and can be followed by the characteristic inspiratory whoop. Complications are frequent: about half of the babies younger than 1-year old who get pertussis need care in the hospital. Of those babies with pertussis who are treated in the hospital, about 1 out of 4 (25%) get pneumonia, 1 out of 100 (1%) will have convulsions, 1 out of 300 (0.3%) will have encephalopathy, and 1 out of 100 (1%) will die.

The best control strategy to prevent pertussis is vaccination. Currently, two types of vaccines against pertussis are in use: the whole-cell vaccines (wP) composed of whole, inactivated bacteria, and the acellular vaccines (aP) consist of purified *B. pertussis* immunogens. With the massive use of the first developed vaccine against the disease, the wP, in the 1950s, the incidence and mortality associated with pertussis fell to very low levels. Reports on safety concerns in the 1970s, however, cast doubt on the wP vaccines' value since they were associated not only with side effects at the injection site but also with serious systemic reactions [9, 10]. These drawbacks contributed to reducing pertussis vaccine acceptance in different countries [10, 11]. The widespread apprehension about wP prompted the development of acellular vaccines containing purified antigenic protein components of *B. pertussis* (two, three, or five immunogens) [12, 13]. Though finally there is no evidence to suggest that wP vaccines cause severe adverse reactions such as brain damage or severe neurological disorder, the aP vaccines are more accepted, especially in industrialized countries where they have gradually superseded the wP formulations. Currently, most of the countries of the EU and the USA use only aP vaccines. The aP formulations restored people's confidence in pertussis-containing vaccines, and infection appeared controlled for several years. Notwithstanding, during the last two decades, the epidemiology of pertussis has changed [14, 15] with several major outbreaks occurring, the incidence of which not only indicated a waning immunity but also demonstrated that the wP vaccines gave children a more lasting immunity than aP [16–18]. Furthermore, the risk of pertussis was increased in schoolchildren, and adolescents vaccinated exclusively with aP compared to those receiving only one wP dose [18, 19]. This difference could result from the weaker immune response induced by aP vaccines characterized mainly by Th2 profiles [20]. In 2015, the Strategic Advisory Group of Experts on immunization expressed concerns regarding the resurgence of pertussis in some industrialized countries despite high aP-vaccine coverage [21]. The switch from wP to aP for primary infant immunization was proposed as at least partially responsible for that resurgence. The World Health Organization (WHO), therefore, recommended considering the switch only if, in the national immunization schedules, large numbers of doses including several boosters could be assured. Countries currently using aP vaccines may continue using them but should consider the need for additional booster doses and strategies to prevent early childhood mortality upon pertussis resurgence.

Besides these recommendations and in order to control the disease in countries that use cellular, acellular, or even mixed vaccine schedules, it is important not only to achieve coverage levels above 95% but also to avoid delays in the application of vaccines [22]. By means of a mathematical model, it was reported that strategies that avoid delays in vaccination have a relevant impact on infant incidences' reduction. It was estimated that the elimination of delays in the primary doses reduces infant incidences by approximately 20% [22]. In the same way, the simultaneous reduction of delays and increased coverage lead to a significant improvement in disease control [22] for those regions where the administration of vaccines was previously deferred for long periods of time.

2. Epidemiology

The maximal risk of pertussis infection and severe morbidity takes place before infants are old enough to have received the primary series of vaccination. [23–25]. In recent years, waning immunity seems to be the main cause for pertussis in adults and adolescents [26–28], and for this reason, these persons constitute a significant reservoir of infection. Evidence from studies of infant pertussis cases indicates that household contacts and carriers are frequently the source of infection, with parents identified as the cause for more than 50% of cases [29]. There has also been a case report documenting nosocomial infection in young infants acquired from health-care workers [30, 31].

Despite a long-standing vaccination program, pertussis remains highly prevalent in many countries [15]. Pertussis is the least well controlled of all vaccine-preventable diseases, and epidemics occur every 3–5 years. During the last decades, multiple epidemics of pertussis took place in many countries including those with high vaccination coverage [14, 15]. In the United States, where aP is used for all vaccination doses since 1996, in 2010–2012, the incidence rate in infants with less than 1 year duplicated those in 2002 (125 vs. 60 per 100,000 inhabitants), and incidence rates were very high not only in infants but also in 7–10-year-old children and adolescents (13–14 years) http://www.cdc.gov/pertussis/outbreaks/trends.html. In 2014, 32,971 cases of pertussis were reported to the Centers for Disease Control and Prevention (CDC). This represents a 15% increase compared to the 28,639 cases reported during 2013. During 2015, a decrease in the number of pertussis cases was reported: 20,762 cases in 2015 compared to 32,971 cases reported during 2014. As in previous years, in 2015, the incidence rate of pertussis in infants exceeded that of all the other age groups. However, the incidence rates in adolescents aged 13–16 years were also high.

Another industrialized country experiencing a notable outbreak is the UK, where, in 2012, 14 infant deaths were reported (Public Health England; cf. https://www.gov.uk/government/publications/whooping-cough-pertussis-statistics, accessed October 2017).

In Australia, the highest annual incidence of notifications (173 cases per 100,000 population) was reported in 2011, with 38,732 notified cases. In the epidemic period 2008–2011, an increase in the reporting of pertussis in children between 3 and 9 years of age was detected. On the other hand, notifications in adolescents and adults decreased compared to previous epidemic periods. In this country, there have been a number of changes introduced to the vaccination schedule over time in an attempt to improve control of pertussis. In this way, acellular pertussis vaccine replaced wP for booster doses in 1997 and for all doses from 1999. In 2003, the aP booster dose at 18 months of age was removed, shifting the first booster dose to 4 years of age.

Outbreaks were also detected in countries where wP vaccines were used. For example, in Argentina, where wP is used for primary series of three doses at 2, 4, and 6 months of age followed by two boosters at 18 months and 6 years old, the number of pertussis reported cases has increased steadily since 2002. In fact, in 2011, reported cases were four times higher than those detected in 2006 (4.1 vs. 16 per 100,000 inhabitants) [32] and 76 deaths were reported in children under 1 year (www.snvs.msal.gov.ar, [32]. Because of this epidemiological situation during 2009, the Ministry of Health recommended vaccination with aP for children at age 11 and for health-care workers in contact with infants under 12 months of age. In 2011, the Argentinean Ministry of Health recommended aP vaccination for household contacts of very-low-birth-weight infants (<1500 g); in 2012, they also offered immunization to all pregnant women after 20 weeks of gestation. Finally, in 2013, the national calendar included the maternal immunization against pertussis during a single pregnancy for each woman, while, in 2016, the recommendation was extended for all pregnancies.

Brazil, other country that uses wP for primary series, reported cases of pertussis from 2007 to 2014 [33]. The annual distribution of confirmed cases demonstrated a significant increase in incidence rate since 2012. Of the 80,068 suspected cases, 32% were confirmed by various criteria. The majority of confirmed cases occurred in infants who were less than 2 months (34.5%) and in infants aged 3–6 months (22.4%). Only 8% of the total confirmed cases was reported in adults >21 years. From the total confirmed cases, 47.2% met only clinical criteria, and 36.6% were confirmed in a laboratory. The overall case fatality rate was 2.1%, reaching 4.7% among infants aged 0–2 months. Of the confirmed cases, 23.1% occurred in subjects who received at least three doses of the pertussis vaccine [33].

These epidemic situations detected in different countries have moved the scientific community and health professionals to seek an understanding of this alarming new situation to identify the causes [34–36], and review and implement new strategies for the control of pertussis [37].

Though several factors apparently contribute to this pertussis-case increase, a consensus exists in identifying, as part of the causes of the epidemic, several factors related to the vaccines currently in use and the vaccination—for example, suboptimal coverage of the three primary doses, noncompliance with vaccination schedule timing (delayed vaccination) [22, 38], the waning of vaccination-conferred immunity [39–41], and the circulation of a resistant bacterial population resulting from the selection pressure exerted by mass vaccination [36]. Probably, the relative contributions of each factor may differ between countries.

To assess the trends of the disease in real time, a reliable and specific pertussis diagnosis is required. Laboratory diagnosis is also important to distinguish between the several etiologic agents of pertussis-like diseases, which involve both viruses and bacteria (i.e., adenovirus, parainfluenza viruses, respiratory syncytial virus, *Mycoplasma pneumoniae*, and *Chlamydophila pneumonia*) [42].

3. Clinical case definition

The clinical case definition used is based on CDC/WHO clinical criteria (www.cdc.gov/ncphi/disss/nndss/casedef/pertussis_current.htm, www.who.int/entity/immunization_monitoring/

diseases/pertussis_surveillance/en/index.html) that refers to a person with a cough illness lasting at least 2 weeks with one of the following symptoms/signs: coughing paroxysms, inspiratory whoop, or post-tussive vomiting. In patients younger than 6 months of age, cyanosis and apneas could also be present, and, for this reason, these symptoms are also included for pertussis clinical diagnosis. The different countries have considered adaptations in clinical criteria including age stratification and cough duration [43].

4. Diagnosis

Although classical pertussis can be diagnosed reliably based on clinical symptoms, infections in infants, older vaccinated children, adolescents, and adults often follow an atypical course. In these cases, the diagnosis of pertussis requires laboratory methods for confirmation. The laboratory criteria for diagnosis are mainly based on isolation of *B. pertussis* from clinical specimen and/or through PCR for *B. pertussis* or serology.

4.1. Culture

The isolation of the etiological agent is the gold standard for pertussis diagnosis. To perform the bacterial isolation, a clinical sample from the nasopharynx should be obtained by aspiration or swabs. Aspirates give better yields than nasopharyngeal swabs though this last could be used, but swabs should be composed of Dacron or nylon if both culture and PCR are to be performed. While cotton swabs are not recommended since they contain substances that could inhibit *B. pertussis* growth, calcium alginate swabs are appropriate only for culture because they inhibit PCRs [44]. Successful recovery of the causative agent depends on a number of factors, including collection and transport conditions of the sample, the stage of disease in which the sample is collected, and the use of antibiotics. *B .pertussis* should be cultivated in Regan Lowe medium and/or Bordet Gengou agar supplemented with defibrinated blood in concentration of 7–15% (**Figure 1**). Addition of the antibiotic cephalexin has been recommended to inhibit growth of contaminating bacteria. However, since cephalexin has been suggested to also inhibit growth of *B. holmesii* [45], plates with and without cephalexin should be used. Incubation periods of up to 10–14 days are recommended for optimal sensitivity. Though *B. pertussis* growth may be retarded, *B. bronchiseptica* usually grows faster (1–3 days), and *B. parapertussis* shows an intermediate growth rate. Growth should be checked daily to prevent overgrowth by contaminating microorganisms.

After growth, *Bordetella* can be detected by Gram staining and identified by biochemical reactions, agglutination with specific sera or PCR. *Bordetella* species can be distinguished biochemically by oxidase, urease, motility, and nitrate reduction.

4.2. PCR assays

Molecular diagnosis methods based on PCR are 2–6 times more sensitive than culture. The sensitivity of the PCR decreases with the time of evolution of the pathology as ocurrs with the microbiological tests. After the 4th week of cough, the amount of bacterial DNA diminishes,

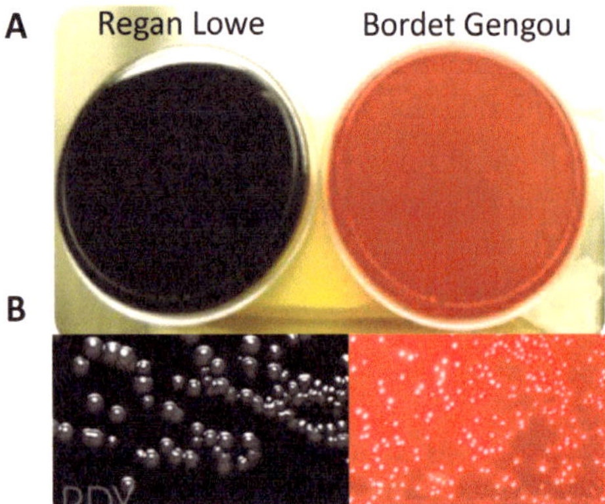

Figure 1. A—Regan low and Bordet Gengou culture media supplemented with 10% v/v sheep blood. B—Growth of *B. pertussis* in Regan Lowe and Bordet Gengou media.

and PCR has optimal sensitivity during the first 3 weeks of cough. As mentioned earlier, the sample of choice is nasopharyngeal aspirate or nasopharyngeal swab.

Extraction and purification of DNA is necessary to limit the action of inhibitors present in samples. There are home methods for the extraction of DNA, which are gradually being replaced by commercial methods. The latter are based on the use of ion exchange resins or magnetic separation using silica particles [46]. Neither of these methods is validated for the extraction of DNA from respiratory samples [46]. There are studies demonstrating that, in general, the different methods are suitable for the extraction of DNA from these samples. The PCR assays have evolved from conventional assays to real-time PCR and from singleplex to multiplex PCR. Conventional PCR employs two different sets of primers that are visualized on agarose gels. The most commonly used target sequences for *B. pertussis* DNA detection are the insertion sequence 481 (*IS*481) and the pertussis toxin promoter region. To detect *B. parapertussis*, primers that hybridize to the insertion sequence *IS*1001 are used. *IS* elements are generally present in multiple copies in genomes, offering excellent targets for highly sensitive PCR detection. *IS*481 and *IS*1001 occur in *B. pertussis* and *B. parapertussis* isolates obtained from humans at copy numbers of 253 and 22, respectively [47, 48]. *IS*481 is also present in *B. holmesii* isolates and in some isolates of *B. bronchiseptica*. These target sequences are also used in real-time PCR assays [49]. In fact, for simultaneous detection of *B. pertussis*, *B. parapertussis*, and *B. holmesii*, a combination of multiplex and singleplex real-time PCR assays targeting IS elements and pertussis toxin sequence has been developed [49].

It is recommended that PCR (conventional or real-time PCR) be used together with the culture. Cultivation of the etiological agent should be performed, especially when an outbreak is suspected.

4.3. Serodiagnosis

Validation and harmonization of serologic methods are still necessary before they can be widely applied as diagnostic tools. Many of the problems associated with serodiagnosis, such as the interference of previous vaccinations or previous infections, cross-reactivity with other *Bordetella* species or perhaps other bacteria, and the variable response to *B. pertussis* antigens should still be overcome. However, in some countries, pertussis serology is currently used for diagnostic purposes [50], in particular, during outbreaks [51].

Bordetella pertussis-specific antibodies can be detected by enzyme-linked immunosorbent assays (ELISAs) or multiplex immunoassays. Assays use purified or mixed antigens, and only pertussis toxin (PTx) is specific for *B. pertussis*. Cross-reactivity with other microbial antigens from other *Bordetella* species could be detected when antibodies against filamentous hemagglutinin (anti-FHA), pertactin (anti-PRN), fimbriae (anti-FIM), and adenylate cyclase (anti-ACT) are measured and, for this reason, the measurement of these antibodies is not recommended for the diagnosis of pertussis. The evaluation of the titers of such antibodies may be used in specific studies [52]. For pertussis diagnosis, only IgG anti-PTx antibody titer evaluation is recommended. IgA and IgM assays lack adequate sensitivity and specificity.

Dual-sample serology based on ≥100% increase in antibody concentration or on ≥50% decrease in antibody concentration is a sensitive and specific method for serological diagnosis [53]. In clinical practice, diagnosis is mostly based on single-sample serology using a single or a more continuous cutoff. The optimal timing for specimen collection is 2–8 weeks following cough onset. For ELISA assays, it is recommended to use a standard serum from WHO [54]. Due to high levels of vaccine-induced IgG-Ptx, single-serum diagnosis is not reliable for 1–3 years after vaccination with Ptx-containing vaccines. If the IgG-Ptx level is below the chosen cutoff, the diagnosis of pertussis can be neither confirmed nor denied, and a second serum obtained at least 2 weeks later and 4–6 weeks after the onset of disease should be investigated. Increases of threefold in paired sera or any increase to a value above the cutoff or absolute values in single sera can then be considered to confirm the diagnosis of pertussis.

4.4. Recommendations for diagnosis testing with suspected pertussis

In neonates and young infants, PCR and/or culture should be performed on nasopharyngeal samples as soon as possible post-onset of symptoms. These methodologies are also recommended in vaccinated children, adolescents, and adults with less than 2 weeks of coughing. For patients older than 11 years with coughing of less than 3 weeks, PCR and IgG-anti-PTx measurement should be performed. The measurement of IgG-anti-PTx is only meaningful for older children/adults, including parents and other household members.

In outbreak situations, PCR and culture should be performed from nasopharyngeal samples and IgG-anti-PTx should be measured in serum samples.

It is important to note here that the microbiological diagnosis for pertussis is more useful during the first 2 weeks of coughing and before starting the antibiotic treatment. PCR assays may effectively be used for pertussis diagnosis from 2–4 weeks of cough. On the other hand, the serological tests are most useful in 2–8 weeks after the onset of cough.

5. Treatment

Early antimicrobial treatment is recommended to reduce transmission and for disease control by protecting close contacts [55]. An antimicrobial can be administered as prophylaxis for close contacts of a person with pertussis if the person has no contraindication to its use.

Individuals with pertussis are infectious from the beginning of the catarrhal period through the first week after the onset of paroxysms and until day 5 after the start of effective antimicrobial treatment.

The macrolide erythromycin has been the antimicrobial of choice for treatment or post-exposure prophylaxis of pertussis [56]. It is usually administered in 4 divided daily doses for 14 days. Unfortunately, erythromycin is accompanied by uncomfortable to distressing side effects that result in poor adherence to the treatment regimen. Two other macrolide agents (azithromycin and clarithromycin) have been shown to be effective against *B. pertussis*. Azithromycin and clarithromycin are more resistant to gastric acid, achieve higher tissue concentrations, and have a longer half-life than erythromycin, allowing less frequent administration (1–2 doses per day) and shorter treatment regimens (5–7 days) [57]. Azithromycin is the preferred antimicrobial for use in infants younger than 1 month of age. The antibiotic doses recommended for infants aged <6 months comprise a regimen of 10 mg/kg per day for 5 days. For patients aged >6 months, 10 mg/kg on day 1, followed by 5 mg/kg per day during the next 4 days is recommended. For adults, 500 mg on day 1 is recommended, followed by 250 mg per day on the following 4 days. The regimen recommended for clarithromycin for infants and children aged >1 month is 15 mg/kg per day in two divided doses each day for 7 days. For adults, 1 g per day in two divided doses for 7 days is recommended. Clarithromycin is not prescribed in infants aged <1 month. Trimethoprim-sulfamethoxazole (TMP-SMZ) in a regimen of two doses a day for 14 days is used as an alternative to a macrolide antibiotic in patients aged >2 months who have contraindication to or cannot tolerate macrolide agents, or who are infected with a macrolide-resistant strain of *B. pertussis*. Resistance of *B. pertussis* to macrolides is rare, and antimicrobial susceptibility testing is not routinely recommended. Testing is appropriate in some circumstances and is recommended when treatment failure is suspected. TMP-SMZ should not be used to treat infants younger than 2 months of age [55].

Because data on the clinical effectiveness of antibiotic treatment against *B. parapertussis* are limited, treatment decisions should be based on clinical judgment [58].

Author details

Daniela Hozbor

Address all correspondence to: hozbor.daniela@gmail.com

Laboratorio VacSal, Instituto de Biotecnología y Biología Molecular (IBBM), Facultad de Ciencias Exactas, Universidad Nacional de La Plata, CCT-CONICET La Plata, La Plata, Argentina

References

[1] Trollfors B, Rabo E. Whooping cough in adults. British Medical Journal (Clinical Research Education). 1981;**283**:696-697

[2] Paisley RD, Blaylock J, Hartzell JD. Whooping cough in adults: An update on a reemerging infection. The American Journal of Medicine. 2012;**125**:141-143

[3] He Q, Viljanen MK, Arvilommi H, Aittanen B, Mertsola J. Whooping cough caused by *Bordetella pertussis* and *Bordetella parapertussis* in an immunized population. JAMA: The Journal of the American Medical Association. 1998;**280**:635-637

[4] Heininger U, Stehr K, Schmitt-Grohe S, Lorenz C, Rost R, Christenson PD, et al. Clinical characteristics of illness caused by Bordetella parapertussis compared with illness caused by Bordetella pertussis. The Pediatric Infectious Disease Journal. 1994;**13**:306-309

[5] Cherry JD, Seaton BL. Patterns of *Bordetella parapertussis* respiratory illnesses: 2008-2010. Clinical Infectious Diseases: An Official Publication of the Infectious Diseases Society of America. 2012;**54**:534-537

[6] Njamkepo E, Bonacorsi S, Debruyne M, Gibaud SA, Guillot S, Guiso N. Significant finding of *Bordetella holmesii* DNA in nasopharyngeal samples from French patients with suspected pertussis. Journal of Clinical Microbiology. 2011;**49**:4347-4348

[7] Spicer KB, Salamon D, Cummins C, Leber A, Marcon MJ. Occurrence of three Bordetella species during an outbreak of cough illness in Ohio: Epidemiology, clinical features, laboratory findings, and antimicrobial susceptibility. The Pediatric Infectious Disease Journal. 2014;**33**(7):e162-e167

[8] Bottero D, Griffith MM, Lara C, Flores D, Pianciola L, Gaillard ME, et al. Bordetella holmesii in children suspected of pertussis in Argentina. Epidemiology and Infection. 2013;**141**:714-717

[9] Jefferson T, Rudin M, DiPietrantonj C. Systematic review of the effects of pertussis vaccines in children. Vaccine. 2003;**21**:2003-2014

[10] Klein NP. Licensed pertussis vaccines in the United States. History and current state. Human Vaccines & Immunotherapeutics. 2014;**10**:2684-2690

[11] Romanus V, Jonsell R, Bergquist SO. Pertussis in Sweden after the cessation of general immunization in 1979. The Pediatric Infectious Disease Journal. 1987;**6**:364-371

[12] Sato H, Sato Y. Protective antigens of *Bordetella pertussis* mouse-protection test against intracerebral and aerosol challenge of *B. Pertussis*. Developments in Biological Standardization. 1985;**61**:461-467

[13] Edwards KM, Karzon DT. Pertussis vaccines. Pediatric Clinics of North America. 1990;**37**:549-566

[14] Clark TA. Changing pertussis epidemiology: Everything old is new again. The Journal of Infectious Diseases. 2014;**209**:978-981

[15] Tan T, Dalby T, Forsyth K, Halperin SA, Heininger U, Hozbor D, et al. Pertussis across the globe: Recent epidemiologic trends from 2000-2013. The Pediatric Infectious Disease Journal. 2015;**34**(9):e222-e232

[16] Klein NP, Bartlett J, Fireman B, Rowhani-Rahbar A, Baxter R. Comparative effectiveness of acellular versus whole-cell pertussis vaccines in teenagers. Pediatrics. 2013;**131**: e1716-e1722

[17] Witt MA, Katz PH, Witt DJ. Unexpectedly limited durability of immunity following acellular pertussis vaccination in preadolescents in a north American outbreak. Clinical Infectious Diseases: An Official Publication of the Infectious Diseases Society of America. 2012;**54**:1730-1735

[18] Sheridan SL, Ware RS, Grimwood K, Lambert SB. Number and order of whole cell pertussis vaccines in infancy and disease protection. JAMA: The Journal of the American Medical Association. 2012;**308**:454-456

[19] Witt MA, Arias L, Katz PH, Truong ET, Witt DJ. Reduced risk of pertussis among persons ever vaccinated with whole cell pertussis vaccine compared to recipients of acellular pertussis vaccines in a large US cohort. Clinical Infectious Diseases: An Official Publication of the Infectious Diseases Society of America. 2013;**56**:1248-1254

[20] Mills KH, Ross PJ, Allen AC, Wilk MM. Do we need a new vaccine to control the re-emergence of pertussis? Trends in Microbiology. 2014;**22**:49-52

[21] Meeting of the Strategic Advisory Group of Experts on immunization, April 2015: conclusions and recommendations. Releve epidemiologique hebdomadaire / Section d'hygiene du Secretariat de la Societe des Nations = Weekly epidemiological record / Health Section of the Secretariat of the League of Nations. 2015;**90**:261-278

[22] Pesco P, Bergero P, Fabricius G, Hozbor D. Mathematical modeling of delayed pertussis vaccination in infants. Vaccine. 2015;**33**:5475-5480

[23] Crowcroft NS, Booy R, Harrison T, Spicer L, Britto J, Mok Q, et al. Severe and unrecognised: Pertussis in UK infants. Archives of Disease in Childhood. 2003;**88**:802-806

[24] Nilsson L, Von Segebaden K, Blennow M, Linde A, Uhnoo I. Whooping cough is a risk to infants. The disease is circulating among adolescents and adults. Läkartidningen. 2013;**110**:1599-1602

[25] Stefanelli P, Buttinelli G, Vacca P, Tozzi AE, Midulla F, Carsetti R, et al. Severe pertussis infection in infants less than 6 months of age: Clinical manifestations and molecular characterization. Human Vaccines & Immunotherapeutics. 2017;**13**:1073-1077

[26] Edwards KM. Unraveling the challenges of pertussis. Proceedings of the National Academy of Sciences of the United States of America. 2014;**111**:575-576

[27] van Boven M, de Melker HE, Schellekens JF, Kretzschmar M. Waning immunity and subclinical infection in an epidemic model: Implications for pertussis in The Netherlands. Mathematical Biosciences. 2000;**164**:161-182

[28] Cherry JD. The role of *Bordetella pertussis* infections in adults in the epidemiology of pertussis. Developments in Biological Standardization. 1997;**89**:181-186

[29] Wiley KE, Zuo Y, Macartney KK, McIntyre PB. Sources of pertussis infection in young infants: A review of key evidence informing targeting of the cocoon strategy. Vaccine. 2013;**31**:618-625

[30] McCall BJ, Tilse M, Burt B, Watt P, Barnett M, McCormack JG. Infection control and public health aspects of a case of pertussis infection in a maternity health care worker. Communicable Diseases Intelligence Quarterly Report. 2002;**26**:584-586

[31] Hospital-acquired pertussis among newborns – Texas, 2004. MMWR Morbidity and Mortality Weekly Report. 2008;**57**:600-603

[32] Romanin V, Agustinho V, Califano G, Sagradini S, Aquino A, Juarez MD, et al. Epidemiological situation of pertussis and strategies to control it: Argentina, 2002-2011. Archivos Argentinos de Pediatria. 2014;**112**:413-420

[33] Guimaraes LM, Carneiro EL, Carvalho-Costa FA. Increasing incidence of pertussis in Brazil: A retrospective study using surveillance data. BMC Infectious Diseases. 2015;**15**:442

[34] He Q, Mertsola J. Factors contributing to pertussis resurgence. Future Microbiology. 2008;**3**:329-339

[35] Jackson DW, Rohani P. Perplexities of pertussis: Recent global epidemiological trends and their potential causes. Epidemiology and Infection. 2014;**142**:672-684

[36] Bart MJ, Harris SR, Advani A, Arakawa Y, Bottero D, Bouchez V, et al. Global population structure and evolution of Bordetella pertussis and their relationship with vaccination. mBio. 2014;**5**:e01074-14

[37] Forsyth K, Plotkin S, Tan T, Wirsing von Konig CH. Strategies to decrease pertussis transmission to infants. Pediatrics. 2015;**135**:e1475-e1482

[38] Gentile A, Bakir J, Firpo V, Caruso M, Lucion MF, Abate HJ, et al. Delayed vaccine schedule and missed opportunities for vaccination in children up to 24 months. A multicenter study. Archivos Argentinos de Pediatria. 2011;**109**:219-225

[39] McGirr A, Fisman DN. Duration of pertussis immunity after DTaP immunization: A meta-analysis. Pediatrics. 2015;**135**:331

[40] Klein NP, Bartlett J, Rowhani-Rahbar A, Fireman B, Baxter R. Waning protection after fifth dose of acellular pertussis vaccine in children. The New England Journal of Medicine. 2012;**367**:1012-1019

[41] Wendelboe AM, Van Rie A, Salmaso S, Englund JA. Duration of immunity against pertussis after natural infection or vaccination. The Pediatric Infectious Disease Journal. 2005;**24**:S58-S61

[42] Wirsing von Konig CH, Rott H, Bogaerts H, Schmitt HJA. Serologic study of organisms possibly associated with pertussis-like coughing. The Pediatric Infectious Disease Journal. 1998;**17**:645-649

[43] Falleiros Arlant LH, de Colsa A, Flores D, Brea J, Avila Aguero ML, Hozbor DF. Pertussis in Latin America: Epidemiology and control strategies. Expert Review of Anti-Infective Therapy. 2014;**12**:1265-1275

[44] Cloud JL, Hymas W, Carroll KC. Impact of nasopharyngeal swab types on detection of *Bordetella pertussis* by PCR and culture. Journal of Clinical Microbiology. 2002;**40**: 3838-3840

[45] Pittet LF, Emonet S, Schrenzel J, Siegrist CA, Posfay-Barbe KM. *Bordetella holmesii*: An under-recognised Bordetella species. The Lancet Infectious Diseases. 2014;**14**:510-519

[46] Riffelmann M, Schmetz J, Bock S. Wirsing von Koenig CH. Preparation of *Bordetella pertussis* DNA from respiratory samples for real-time PCR by commercial kits. European Journal of Clinical Microbiology & Infectious Diseases: Official Publication of the European Society of Clinical Microbiology. 2008;**27**:145-148

[47] McLafferty MA, Harcus DR, Hewlett EL. Nucleotide sequence and characterization of a repetitive DNA element from the genome of *Bordetella pertussis* with characteristics of an insertion sequence. Journal of General Microbiology. 1988;**134**:2297-2306

[48] van der Zee A, Agterberg C, van Agterveld M, Peeters M, Mooi FR. Characterization of IS1001, an insertion sequence element of *Bordetella parapertussis*. Journal of Bacteriology. 1993;**175**:141-147

[49] Tatti KM, Tondella ML. Utilization of multiple real-time PCR assays for the diagnosis of Bordetella spp. in clinical specimens. Methods in Molecular Biology. 2013;**943**:135-147

[50] Guiso N, Berbers G, Fry NK, He Q, Riffelmann M. Wirsing von Konig CH. What to do and what not to do in serological diagnosis of pertussis: Recommendations from EU reference laboratories. European Journal of Clinical Microbiology & Infectious Diseases: Official Publication of the European Society of Clinical Microbiology. 2011;**30**:307-312

[51] Rodgers L, Martin SW, Cohn A, Budd J, Marcon M, Terranella A, et al. Epidemiologic and laboratory features of a large outbreak of pertussis-like illnesses associated with cocirculating *Bordetella holmesii* and *Bordetella pertussis* – Ohio, 2010-2011. Clinical Infectious Diseases: An Official Publication of the Infectious Diseases Society of America. 2013;**56**:322-331

[52] Meade BD, Lynn F, Reed GF, Mink CM, Romani TA, Deforest A, et al. Relationships between functional assays and enzyme immunoassays as measurements of responses to acellular and whole-cell pertussis vaccines. Pediatrics. 1995;**96**:595-600

[53] Simondon F, Iteman I, Preziosi MP, Yam A, Guiso N. Evaluation of an immunoglobulin G enzyme-linked immunosorbent assay for pertussis toxin and filamentous hemagglutinin in diagnosis of pertussis in Senegal. Clinical and Diagnostic Laboratory Immunology. 1998;**5**:130-134

[54] Xing D, Wirsing von Konig CH, Newland P, Riffelmann M, Meade BD, Corbel M, et al. Characterization of reference materials for human antiserum to pertussis antigens by an international collaborative study. Clinical and Vaccine Immunology: CVI. 2009;**16**:303-311

[55] Tiwari T, Murphy TV, Moran J. Recommended antimicrobial agents for the treatment and postexposure prophylaxis of pertussis: 2005 CDC guidelines. MMWR Recommendations and reports: Morbidity and Mortality Weekly Report Recommendations and Reports / Centers for Disease Control. 2005;**54**:1-16

[56] Bergquist SO, Bernander S, Dahnsjo H, Sundelof B. Erythromycin in the treatment of pertussis: A study of bacteriologic and clinical effects. The Pediatric Infectious Disease Journal. 1987;**6**:458-461

[57] Aoyama T, Sunakawa K, Iwata S, Takeuchi Y, Fujii R. Efficacy of short-term treatment of pertussis with clarithromycin and azithromycin. The Journal of Pediatrics. 1996;**129**: 761-764

[58] Hoppe JE, Tschirner T. Comparison of media for agar dilution susceptibility testing of *Bordetella pertussis* and *Bordetella parapertussis*. European Journal of Clinical Microbiology & Infectious Diseases: Official Publication of the European Society of Clinical Microbiology. 1995;**14**:775-779

Chapter 3

Clinical Experiences in Pertussis in a Population with High Vaccination Rate

Filumena Maria da Silva Gomes,
Maria Helena Valente,
Ana Maria de Ulhôa Escobar and
Sandra Josefina Ferraz Ellero Grisi

Additional information is available at the end of the chapter

http://dx.doi.org/10.5772/intechopen.75684

Abstract

Infection caused by *Bordetella pertussis* in young infants can lead to severe illness and death. Several countries with good pertussis vaccine coverage, above 90%, had outbreaks of this disease from 2010, including Brazil. One of the strategies to reduce the transmission of pertussis to young infants, especially below 6 months of age, is the introduction of Tdap vaccination in pregnant women between 27 and 36 weeks of gestation. Vaccination of pregnant women with Tdap is an emergency measure to reduce hospitalizations and deaths from pertussis in young infants, especially those younger than 3 months of age, which is the population group where the most frequent serious illness occurs. Passive immunity to pertussis in these newborns is temporary, lasting less than 6 months, and there is discussion in the literature of its interference with maternal immunity and immunity of young infants to other vaccines. The acquired immunity to pertussis, both by natural disease and by vaccines, is temporary, and it is known that the immune response to the acellular vaccine is smaller and less durable than the whole-cell vaccine. New strategies for pertussis control should be developed to better cope with this disease overall.

Keywords: pertussis, *Bordetella pertussis*, whole-cell pertussis vaccines, acellular pertussis vaccines, maternal pertussis vaccination, passive protection, infants, vaccine effectiveness, whooping cough

1. Introduction

Whooping cough is mentioned in medical literature since 1540, in the pre-vaccine era, when the incidence of the disease ranged from 100 to 200 cases per 100,000 people [1, 2].

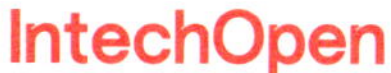

This same incidence is observed nowadays in many developing countries and also in some high-income countries among children under 1 year of age. The vaccine age begins in the 1940s with the whole-cell pertussis vaccines (wP vaccines) and in 1992 with acellular pertussis vaccines (aP vaccines) in developed countries, with a marked decrease in the number of sick individuals as well as in the number of hospitalizations. Despite this, there has been an increase in the incidence and deaths due to pertussis in infants fewer than 6 months of age between 1980 and 2010 in the USA, in Europe, and in many other countries [1–5]. Whooping cough is a highly infectious disease caused by *Bordetella pertussis* and, more rarely, by *Bordetella parapertussis, B. bronchiseptica,* or *B. holmesii.* It is the most ill-controlled vaccine-preventable bacterial disease in countries with high vaccination coverage, in which disease peaks occur every 3–5 years. Although routine childhood vaccination has produced a substantial reduction in the number of cases, it continues to cause high morbidity and mortality in children in countries across the globe [6–8]. In developed countries with pertussis vaccination coverage above 90–95%, such as the USA, the UK, several European countries, and Australia, pertussis has manifested in children under 6 months of age when they have not yet completed their primary series and in adolescents and adults who lost their immunity induced by the vaccine (the last booster is given at the age of 5 years). Young infants present atypical and potentially serious conditions, with about 50% of the cases leading to hospitalizations and often even to death, while adolescents and adults also present atypical but mild symptomatology, and as a result, the individual is often mistakenly diagnosed with other infections of the upper respiratory tract [2, 3, 9, 10]. The causes of the decreasing immunity to pertussis are varied: from the primary vaccine failure due to bacterial adaptations to the failure of the vaccine to eliminate the bacteria from the carriers' organism and thereby prevent transmission to the dropping of protective antibodies. The duration of protection of the acellular vaccines is approximately 3 years, with 85% efficacy, and the risk of contracting the disease increases by 1.33 times each year after the last dose of the vaccine. Therefore, the vaccine protects against the disease, but not against bacterial colonization and its consequent transmission. Loss of vaccine-derived protection over time and increased circulation of *B. pertussis* lead to increased susceptibility of adolescents and adults. As a result, whooping cough is often reported as a cause of persistent cough in adolescents and adults [6, 11–14]. The variation in the notification of the age group affected by pertussis can be explained in part by a growing recognition of the less typical manifestations of the disease in adolescents and adults and by severe cases in young infants. It can also be explained by the development of more sensitive laboratory tests and by a more sensitive and extended healthcare surveillance to cover all life periods [15–17]. Outbreaks in areas of high vaccination coverage demand a review of vaccination strategies. It is necessary to take into account adolescent and adult transmitters, as well as health professionals and pregnant women. In order to better assess changes in epidemiology over time and to optimize disease control, it is important to improve whooping cough surveillance, from clinical recognition of the disease to laboratory diagnosis [18]. In 2013, according to the WHO estimates, pertussis caused about 63,000 deaths in children under 5 years of age, although there is considerable uncertainty about these estimates in view of the scarcity of reliable surveillance data, especially in developing countries [16, 19]. In 2014, pertussis global vaccination coverage was estimated at 86%, considering adherence to the vaccine primary series of three doses. A change in age distribution of the disease for older children and certain age groups (adolescents and young adults) has been reported in recent years in some high-income countries, in particular where aP vaccines have replaced wP vaccines in primary series and booster doses [15, 16]. High vaccination coverage needs to be maintained in order to ensure protection of newborns and young infants, the two groups most likely to show the most severe symptoms and who have not yet started or did not complete their primary series of vaccines. The recent shortage of pertussis vaccine in Europe and elsewhere represents a considerable challenge for maintaining such coverage [18]. It is estimated that the incidence of whooping cough is actually 6–9 times higher than the reported cases, which in 2016, according to the WHO, were 139,535 cases. The unfamiliarity with the disease and its incorrect diagnosis seem to be particularly common among adolescents and adults, due to its atypical clinical presentation. Persistent cough is often the only sign of the disease, and this signal can be attributed to many other conditions and is generally not correlated to whooping cough; so, diagnostic is not performed. On the other hand, the search for specific antibodies in respiratory secretions of patients with chronic cough usually comes as negative. Only serology will identify the cases, and, in turn, serology may not be able to differentiate current active cases from recent cases. The actual incidence of pertussis remains unknown, because data collection varies greatly between countries, which affect the interpretation of trends. There are also variations in the diagnostic methods for laboratory confirmation, in the definition of a case of pertussis and the clinical diagnosis itself [18, 20, 21]. In addition to all the difficulties of data collection, there is still the issue of high contagiousness of the disease, even among vaccinated individuals. A study carried out on vaccinated children, aged 1–5 years, in a preschool class, who had contact with a pertussis case, observed attack rates approaching 50%. This shows the importance of diagnostic investigations even in vaccinated children. The clini cal condition will also highly depend on the history of each child, which emphasizes the seriousness of the matter [22].

2. Whooping cough: current situation

There is no consensus as to why the number of pertussis cases has increased in countries with high vaccination coverage. The reasons range from improvements in diagnosis, earlier diagnosis, and more accurate surveillance. These changes have led to an increase in the number of reported cases, but there is also evidence of increased circulation of the bacteria in the population. There are several other explanations for increased epidemics: changes in circulating pertussis virulence, vaccine failure against new bacteria, vaccine failure to block transmission of infection, decreased adherence to vaccination, rapid loss of immunity in adolescents and adults due to the vaccine or due to the disease itself over time, making the vaccinated individuals susceptible, and also the increase of susceptible individuals in the population [10, 17, 23–25].

2.1. Loss of immunity

Neither vaccination nor disease induces long-term protection against pertussis. Loss of protection occurs from 4 to 12 years after the last dose of vaccine and from 7 to 20 years after an episode of disease. The duration of protection of the whole-cell vaccine corresponds to that of the natural infection [3, 25].

The protection evoked by the vaccine tends to get lost over time. Predicted time of the drop of antibody protective levels after vaccination to pre-vaccine levels varies according to different antigens: 15.3 years for pertactin, 11 years for fimbria types 2 and 3, 5 years for pertussis toxin (PT), and 9.5 years for filamentous hemagglutinin. Adolescent vaccination has a good cost-benefit, since it leads to a significant reduction in costs with the disease, but yet not all developed countries provide the booster dose for individuals aged between 10 and 17 years. There is evidence that immunization of adolescents also does not provide long-term protection, which may lead to the risk of adults and elderly people being more affected by infection. This raises the issue that adults should also receive booster doses, since adolescents and adults only have protection for a few years, and should receive booster doses every 10 years [20].

The antibodies to pertactin are correlated to the protection of the disease, but nowadays there is an increase of non-pertactin producing *B. pertussis* strains. In developed countries that use the acellular vaccine (which has pertactin as one of its components), loss of immunity may occur, as well as failure to prevent colonization by pertussis. However, other components of the vaccine (pertussis toxin, filamentous hemagglutinin, or fimbriae) also seem to prevent symptomatic pertussis [26].

2.2. Pertussis genetic changes

Genetic changes in *B. pertussis* may be one of the factors that have contributed to the recent reappearance of whooping cough. In the USA, isolated cases of *Bordetella pertussis* without pertactin have increased from 14% in 2010 to 85% in 2012. The effectiveness of the acellular vaccine appears to remain the same, but surveillance for the adaptations and mutations of the bacteria must be enhanced, as new genotypes have been reported [26, 27].

2.3. Current situation around the world

In the USA, notable increases in pertussis disease occurred in 2004 (25,827 cases, 27 deaths), in 2010 (27,550 cases, 27 deaths), and, more recently, in 2012, when more than 41,000 cases and 18 deaths have been reported, the largest number of cases in the USA since 1959. In addition, the epidemiological characteristics of whooping cough have changed in recent years with an increased load of disease among fully vaccinated children and adolescents [28].

In 2012 when whooping cough was epidemic in the USA, there was an incidence of 103 cases per 100,000 inhabitants in Vermont. These evidences suggest a resurgence of pertussis in the USA [3, 26].

According to the WHO SAGE pertussis working group report in April 2014 [3], the data from the USA suggest a decrease in immunity after aP vaccine replaced wP, but no impact was observed on overall infant mortality. It also indicates the limited duration of the protection for pertussis in adolescents, pointing to the need for booster vaccination in adolescents who received the aP vaccine compared to those who had at least one dose of wP. There was no resurgence of the disease in Canada, but the periodic cycle had a higher peak in 2012 than in the previous two cycles. An increase in reported cases was limited to certain regions and happened over short periods. In general, the situation in the country is very heterogeneous with multiple causes for increase in pertussis cases (low vaccine coverage, decreasing immunity, previous wP vaccine with low efficacy), but there is no evidence that aP has contributed to the most recent increase in cases. The data suggest that the immunity induced by aP vaccines decreases before the booster dose of adolescence. Therefore, it can be concluded that the timing of adolescent's vaccination is important and that the age in which the third booster is commonly ministered (14–16 years old) may be too late.

In Brazil, a country that still uses wP vaccines, national vaccination coverage in infants under 1 year of age with DTP3 (diphtheria-tetanus-pertussis) vaccine was high (>95%) between 2001 and 2011. From 2006 to 2012, the number of municipalities with coverage above 95% decreased from 83 to 55%, resulting in a heterogeneous coverage throughout the country. The causes for the decline were mainly operational issues due to supply and social problems. In Brazil, the number of pertussis cases increased from 2001 to 2012, with a large increase in morbidity and mortality among infants under 1 year old. This increase was attributed in part to improvements in surveillance sensitivity. Between 2007 and 2012, 51% of reported cases of whooping cough in children under 6 months of age did not receive any dose of vaccine, 37% received only one dose against whooping cough, and 12% received 2 or more doses. The majority of deaths, 342 (97%), occurred in children younger than 1 year of age. The increase in fatal cases among children under 6 months of age led the country to introduce the aP vaccine in pregnant women and also to recommend a cocooning strategy. The recurrence of the natural cycle, the drop in vaccination coverage, and the increase in laboratory tests may be responsible for the increase in the number of cases. There is no evidence of diminishing immunity, as cases are predominant in young infants not yet immunized, supported by the fact that the increase is not observed in older age groups, and the change in disease activity does not exceed what would normally be expected in epidemic cycles [3, 29].

In Chile, the quality of data was improved in 2012, since the laboratory methods were previously not ideal. The resurgence of whooping cough observed in 2011 and 2012 was preceded by a drop in vaccine coverage and thus may be partly linked to this fall [3]. In Cuba, the notification is based only on the clinical definition, without laboratory confirmation. The country's data is therefore not comparable with data from other countries, thereby limiting its usefulness [3]. In Mexico, the data quality has serious limitations, and the sensitivity of the surveillance system is low. The increase in cases may be related to the low and heterogeneous vaccination coverage. The use of a more sensitive laboratory method (PCR) may explain the recent increase in cases, an idea supported by the dissociation of the total infant cases from whooping cough and infant mortality in 2012 [3]. In the European Union (EU), 40,727 cases of whooping cough were notified in 29 countries in 2014. The reporting rate was 9.1 cases per 100,000 inhabitants, higher than in 2013 but lower than in the epidemic year of 2012 [18]. Germany reported 12,339 cases (15.3 cases per 100,000 inhabitants) in 2014. Rates were highest among children under 1 year of age (51.6 cases per 100,000 individuals), followed by 10–14 years (24.4 per 100,000) and 15–19 years (19.7 per 100,000). The German data is of good quality; therefore, the hypothesis of resurgence of the disease can be discarded. A low overall incidence and low numbers of hospitalizations are observed despite the years of recurrent outbreaks. The increase in incidence may be due to the greater number of serological tests in adolescents [3, 18]. Spain has had a higher mortality rate and hospitalization for whooping cough in children under 3 months of age in 2010 (142.55/100,000) [30–32]. The situation in Denmark is stable, with an observed increase in cases occurring by natural recurrent cycles of the disease and by the use of serological diagnosis. Denmark is the only country with the exclusive use of monovalent aP vaccine: primary immunization begins at 3 months of age, followed by doses at 5 and 12 months. Since 2004, the total number of reported cases has remained relatively stable since the introduction of the aP vaccine, contrary to what has been reported by other countries that have used long-term aP vaccines [3, 5]. The observed epidemiology of Finland is explained by naturally occurring cycles. The situation is stable; no statistically significant change in trends is identified after 2003–2004. Since the aP vaccine was introduced in 2005, the time elapsed is still short to allow observation of possible resurgence of the disease due to the decrease in aP-related immunity. In France, there was no resurgence of the disease, with the aP vaccine being used in the past 10 years with a high coverage. Available data suggest a recent increase in incidence in the age range between 5 and 10, which may reflect an increasing decrease in protection in cohorts exclusively vaccinated with aP. New strategies, such as adult reinforcement and cocooning, have not had a major impact, and their level of implementation remains low [3]. The incidence of pertussis in Belgium at all ages was estimated from 24.2 to 30.8 per 100,000 individuals in 2014. In a study with identification of *B. pertussis* with real-time PCR, the culture of these cases was positive in 30%. In this same study, 60% of the cases were positive in serology with anti-PT antibodies, two serology samples were required, and rare cases were positive for both methods, with which it was demonstrated that diagnosis may require both microbiological and immunological methods [3, 25, 33]. In Portugal, there was a significant increase in incidence in infants under 1 year of age, suggesting a true resurgence of the disease, although the increased incidence may also be associated with the increased use of the PCR test. Pertussis infant mortality was very high in 2012, while mortality from the period 2000 to 2011 was similar to that of other countries. There is likely underreporting in the older age groups. The whole-cell vaccine was replaced by acellular vaccine in 2006. In Sweden there has been no resurgence of pertussis to date, and there have been no major outbreaks since 2004. There has been a successive reduction in the overall incidence of whooping cough since the reintroduction of the vaccine against pertussis after a 17-year period without the vaccine [3]. In the UK, evidence suggests a resurgence of whooping cough. Although the incidence has declined in the last 20 years, there has been no interruption of the natural epidemic cycle, which happens every 3–4 years. A real increase over the natural cycle was observed in infants younger than 3 months of age in 2011 and 2012. An increase in reported cases, hospitalizations, and the number of deaths in young infants was observed. The actual resurgence of pertussis was recorded 7 years after the introduction of the aP vaccine, coinciding with the peak of the natural epidemic cycle [3]. In Eastern European countries, there have been several outbreaks, whose incidence varied from 0.01 to as high as 96 per 100,000 inhabitants. The highest index was found in Estonia [34]. The data available in Israel do not provide clear evidence of the resurgence of pertussis.

Possible explanations for the increase in child cases include greater awareness of whooping cough and the availability of better laboratory tests. Vaccination coverage is high in Israel, which has been using aP (ranging from 3 to 5 components) for the past 7 years [3]. Incidence data for children under 6 years of age in Japan were highest in 2000. The most recent data (2010) show an increase in cases of adults over 20 years. This increase was surprisingly not reflected in young infants, and only a small increase can be observed among older children. No data were obtained concerning hospitalizations and deaths related to whooping cough in Japan. There is no evidence of resurgence, although data are limited [35]. The quality of the data is good in Singapore, and there is no evidence of the resurgence of whooping cough [3]. The data does not allow drawing conclusions about the sudden increase in pertussis in 2007 among those unimmunized or with incomplete immunization, which may be due to the introduction of PCR or whether it was a real increase with case duplication in 2007. Despite the two peaks in 2007 and 2011, the overall incidence was low. The recent rise in whooping cough began shortly after moving from wP to aP vaccine in 2006. Data quality is limited in Thailand, since cases are underreported and there is a low sensitivity of the surveillance system. There is no evidence of a resurgence of whooping cough: incidence remained low between 2009 and 2014. Thailand uses only wP vaccination [3, 36]. In Australia, there was a resurgence of whooping cough between 2008 and 2012 in children under 10 years of age, in particular at 2–4 and 7–9 age ranges. Pertussis is an important public health issue in Australia, with continuous increases observed over a long period of time. The increase was observed at first in adults, related to the availability of serological tests, and then in adolescents, which was related to a history of low coverage of vaccines. More recently, increase of pertussis was observed in younger children, consistent with declining immunity in the context of increased availability and use of tests. Withdrawal of the booster dose in early childhood (at 18 months of age) appears to have made an important contribution to the resurgence of the disease in children aged 2–4 years, with decreasing immunity after the last dose of acellular vaccine at 6 months. The 18-month vaccine was reintroduced in 2015. As in the USA, Australia had large increases of the disease in children over 6 years of age [3, 37, 38].

There are few publications on pertussis in Africa, and most of them do not contain surveillance data and epidemiological trends. In addition we have lack of laboratories capable of adequate diagnosis [39]. Based on the WHO data, the number of cases of pertussis in Africa decreased from 2000 to 2010, except in 2011, when an increase occurred [40]. The WHO in 2016 reported 139,535 cases of pertussis in the world, and in Africa we had only 1425 reported cases [21]. Nigeria, on the other hand, had a peak in whooping cough activity in 2009, reporting the second largest number of cases worldwide, and the diagnosis was made primarily clinical as there are few laboratories for the research [40]. In some African countries, wP vaccine coverage is very low, as measured in Chad (22%), Equatorial Guinea (33%), Gabon (45%), Nigeria (47%), Liberia 49%), Ethiopia (51%), Central African Republic (54%), Guinea (59%), Cote d'Ivoire (62%), and Cameroon (68%) [40]. The WHO African Regional Office (AFRO) is working on reducing missed opportunities for vaccination in 20 priority countries representing 30% (5.9 million) of the unvaccinated or partially vaccinated global birth cohort [41].

Country-specific data provided no evidence of a widespread resurgence of whooping cough globally. The increase in the number of pertussis cases observed in recent years has been attributed to cyclical patterns in most countries, probably amplified by increased disease awareness, increased global laboratory tests, and increased sensitivity of diagnostic methods, as well as by the use of PCR amplification. Recurrent natural cycles may be more visible in countries where surveillance is more sensitive and where disease control in recent years has generally been good.

Data from only five of these countries (Australia, Chile, Portugal, the USA, and the UK) supported the hypothesis of a real resurgence in pertussis-related morbidity in recent years compared to previous periods of time. Only one country that used wP vaccine against pertussis, Chile, reported a resurgence. For the time being, the increase in cases can be attributed to a sustained decrease in vaccine coverage, to variable coverage at the district level, to changes in surveillance practices, as well as to problems with the specificity of diagnostic tests. The increase in infant cases was noteworthy and associated with increased disease mortality. However, since this was based on fluorescent antibody test data alone (which is known to have problems with specificity), more data will be needed for a better characterization of the problem [3, 39].

3. Vaccination and control strategies

There is a wide variety of vaccine calendars in the world. By 2015, 86% of children worldwide (116.1 million) received three doses of diphtheria, tetanus, and pertussis (DTP) vaccines. However, to reach coverage of 95% or more, 13.5 million unvaccinated children should be vaccinated annually, and an additional 6 million children with incomplete vaccination should complete the timeline. Restricted access and missed opportunities for vaccination remain a challenge worldwide, as well as for middle- and upper-income countries [41].

3.1. Newborns

The increased incidence of whooping cough in countries with high vaccine coverage is alarming, with rates only previously seen in 1950. The protection of newborns is urgently needed, especially during the period between birth and the first dose of the vaccine [10].

Vaccination in newborns is not an option at the present time, both due to the immaturity of the immune system of the newborn and its weak response to the vaccine. Besides these factors, the vaccine against pertussis may also interfere with the newborn's response to the hepatitis B vaccine. For the protection of the newborn, we currently can resort to three related strategies: cocooning, booster schedule, and vaccination of pregnant women [10, 42].

3.2. Children: primary vaccination and booster schedule

The WHO recommends three doses of vaccine in the primary series, the first dose being given at 6 weeks of age (at the latest at 8 weeks of age). The second dose should be given 4–8 weeks after the first one. The last dose should be given at 6 months of age or at any opportunity after. Delaying the third dose may reduce protection against severe illness in the first year of life. A booster dose is recommended after 1 year of age, preferably in the second year of life, 6 months after the primary vaccination scheme. In countries that use aP vaccine, protection diminishes before the age of 6 years old, whereas those who use wP offer a protection that lasts for 6 years or more. A second booster dose should be given from 4 to 6 years of age for both vaccines [16, 43].

National programs currently administering wP vaccination should continue to use wP vaccines for the primary vaccination series. National programs currently using the aP vaccine may continue to use this vaccine but should consider the need for additional booster doses and additional strategies, such as maternal immunization in case of pertussis resurgence. Only the aP vaccine can be administered in individuals from the age of 7 onward. Vaccination at this age must be based on cost-effectiveness mindset, since the priority is always to maintain high vaccination coverage in the first years of life [16].

3.3. Adolescents and adults: booster schedule

The acellular vaccine was introduced in 1992 in the American calendar, and in 1997 it was already part of the entire childhood calendar (2, 4, 6, and 15 months and 4–6 years). In 2006, a booster dose was introduced at 11–12 years old. Despite this, there was a large outbreak in 2012 in children vaccinated with the acellular vaccine, probably due to the loss of immunity, lower immune response induced by the aP, increased awareness and notification, as well as improved diagnostic techniques, and possibly genetic alterations of the bacteria [26].

One of the reasons for the increase in pertussis is the loss of immunity induced by the vaccine or by infection among adolescents and adults. This leads to the discussion about the need for changes in the vaccine calendars of adolescents and adults. In countries with high vaccination coverage, there has also been an increase in pertussis cases in adolescents and adults in recent years, which is one of the causes of the onset of diseases in young infants, so a vaccine booster in adolescence and adulthood is recommended in order to reduce the spread of the disease among young infants [20].

The duration of immunity of the wP vaccine is 4–12 years, and the aP protection begins to diminish after 4–5 years. This led to the need of a booster dose in the adolescence (from 8 to 11 years), because adolescents present low levels of antibodies, which increase later in life (from 12 to 15 years) due to natural infection [44].

Although a booster dose in adolescence has been shown to decrease the disease in adolescents, this is generally not recommended as a means of controlling disease in infants. Introduction of reinforcements in adolescents and/or in adults should only be done after evaluation of local epidemiology [16, 43]. Adult vaccination in most countries with high vaccination coverage is done with dT, and even when done with dTap, as in the USA, this occurs in only 14.2% of adults who have done so in the last 7 years [45].

One of the risk factors associated with pertussis in young infants is the presence of a household contact, usually parents, siblings, or caregivers, with a cough for 5 days or more [46].

3.4. Pregnant women: booster doses

One of the strategies to reduce the transmission of pertussis to young infants, especially less than 6 months of age, is the introduction of Tdap vaccination in pregnant women between 27 and 36 weeks of gestation in all pregnancies (not just the first one). Vaccination of the pregnant woman is most effective when administered 28 days or more before delivery, when a greater number of antibodies are transferred to the fetus. No adverse events were reported for the mother or the newborn with this measure, except for a small significant increase in chorioamnionitis seen by Kharbanda in 2014 [47–50]. The transplacental transfer of vaccine-induced antibodies from the pregnant woman to the fetus before birth and through maternal breastfeeding after birth is the basis of the prenatal immunization [19]. If the mother is vaccinated with the aP vaccine during pregnancy, her maternal antibodies against pertussis will also be transferred to the newborn through breast milk [46].

In 2012, vaccination of pregnant women in the third trimester of pregnancy was instituted by the American Centers for Disease Control and Prevention (CDC), regardless of their vaccination status, due to the loss of immunity a few months after booster vaccination. Several studies have attested the safety of dTap use in pregnant women [51, 52]. These studies showed that women vaccinated before pregnancy had less than 50% detectable antibodies against pertussis during gestation, which led to the adoption of the measure of vaccinating the woman at each gestation, regardless of her previous vaccination status [10, 53]. Vaccination in pregnant women between 27 and 36 weeks is more effective for the prevention of pertussis in young infants than vaccination in the second trimester of pregnancy. On the other hand, it is known that the vaccine given at the beginning of this period of 27–31 weeks is more effective in reducing pertussis in young infants. Efforts should be made for adequate vaccination schedule during prenatal consultations. Vaccination of 27–36 weeks is 85% more effective than Tdap postpartum vaccination [12, 51].

In the UK, vaccination was introduced in 2012 for pregnant woman between 28 and 32 weeks. In 2016, the country began recommending vaccination between 16 and 32 weeks, in order to improve the chance of vaccination to protect preterm infants, as well as to improve the level of maternal antibodies at birth. Later, vaccination during pregnancy protects the mother from developing the disease, giving some degree of protection to the newborn. Some studies have shown that women who were vaccinated after 32 weeks of pregnancy did not have the best level of passive protection for the newborn. In Belgium, the orientation for pregnant women is from 24 to 32 weeks of gestation [19, 25, 54, 55].

The timing of pregnant women vaccination is still controversial, with recent studies recommending it in the second trimester of pregnancy, while previous studies advocated for the third trimester [10, 52].

The recommendation of vaccination in pregnant women has expanded to several countries, such as Argentina, Belgium, Brazil, Colombia, El Salvador, Mexico, New Zealand, Australia, Switzerland, Ireland, the Czech Republic, Israel, Spain, and Greece [19].

It is known that the transfer of maternal antibodies to the newborn can interfere with the response of young infants to their own vaccination [56, 57], a phenomenon called blunting. This phenomenon depends on the type of vaccine antibody: the PT antibody increases after primary immunization, but the FHA antibody decreases in infants born from mothers vaccinated during pregnancy [19, 58, 59]. A study showed that the level of antibodies in the newborn and infants of mothers vaccinated for pertussis was adequate and protective, although their levels were slightly lower after the first three doses of the vaccine, and there was no difference in antibody levels after the first booster in the second year of life [10]. Monitoring the immunity of children vaccinated or not should be done regardless of age, in order to understand the long-term impact and the real significance of these immunological findings [19].

Prenatal vaccination induces protection against pertussis by producing high levels of antibodies, which are transferred to the fetus. This strategy will protect newborns when they are vulnerable to the disease, which happens mainly in the period before they complete their primary vaccination schedule with all three doses of the vaccine [19].

Vaccination in pregnant women is the most cost-effective strategy for disease prevention in young infants and unvaccinated newborns. It is more effective to vaccinate the pregnant mother than to vaccinate those interacting with the baby. The vaccine should be given in the second or third trimester of pregnancy, at least 15 days before delivery. This strategy should be adopted in countries with high or increasing morbidity and mortality of young infants due to pertussis [16, 60].

3.5. Caregivers: cocooning strategy

The cocooning strategy consists of vaccinating the whole family and intimate contacts of the newborn, in addition to vaccination of the pregnant woman. It is important to remember that the vaccine takes 2 weeks to raise the antibodies to protective levels; therefore, the newborn is exposed to the transmission of the pertussis during this critical period [20]. Vaccination of household members is effectively provided as it is performed in a timely manner [16]. All caregivers of young infants (who feed, dress, and bathe them regularly) should also be considered for vaccination [46]. It is necessary to achieve adherence by all of those in contact with the newborn or young infant, in order to obtain the effectiveness of the cocooning strategy. It is important to note that the mother accepts this initiative better than the father of the child and other relatives tend to accept it even more rarely [20].

In an American study of 115 young infants with severe pertussis, 72% had previously had contact with adults or children over 11 years of age who showed acute cough for 5 days or more, referred to in the last month. This contact was often with the mother. The fact that infants received a dose of aP did not protect them from the disease [46]. The route of contamination was usually through a member of the family [6].

It has been observed that infants and young infants with older siblings are also at increased risk for pertussis. Each older sibling of the young infant increases the chance of having pertussis 1.5 times more, speaking in favor of the hypothesis that the source of contamination is the older sibling [12].

The American CDC recommends vaccination with a dose of Tdap for every adult and adolescent who have contact or who live with infants younger than 12 months of age [50]. Chile also adopted this strategy in 2011 with a significant impact: there was an 84% reduction in infant mortality when comparing cocooning strategy with no action taken [3].

Cocooning doses may reduce the serious morbidity of the infant, but timing is crucial, and the overall impact and cost-effectiveness may vary between countries and situations. The advantages of cocooning are better acceptance of vaccination in the postpartum period than during pregnancy, accessibility to the whole family, and the opportunity for health education. Disadvantages are the slow response to produce immunity to protect the newborn and logistical and economic issues. In addition, the challenges to implementing cocooning strategies include parental refusal, political hardship, logistical issues, and cultural issues. The cost–benefit ratio of cocooning is lower than maternal immunization, since it requires only one dose, whereas the cocooning strategy requires at least two doses for both parents [3, 61].

Vaccination of pregnant women is likely to be the most cost-effective additional strategy to prevent pertussis disease in young infants and appears to be more effective and favorable than the cocooning strategy.

3.6. Healthcare professionals: booster schedule

In countries that have implemented pertussis vaccination for adults, vaccination of healthcare workers should be given priority, but there is no evidence that this decreases the acquisition or transmission of the disease but otherwise avoids nosocomial disease transmitted to newborns and young infants. Health professionals in contact with pregnant women, parturients, newborns, and young infants should also be prioritized. New studies are needed to assess the real impact of this measure [16, 44, 62].

4. Conclusions

Health education programs are needed to improve adherence to the pertussis immunization programs. Scientific divulgation of the disease and its prevention strategies are fundamental. Vaccination, especially for pregnant women and young infants, must also be publicized, as well as the discussion for incorporation of the vaccine against pertussis into the vaccination programs for adolescents, adults, and the elderly.

Vaccination for pertussis has had a major impact in reducing the overall burden of the disease, with a general reduction in its incidence and, in particular, a reduction in infant mortality. Nevertheless, the cyclic and recurrent patterns of whooping cough are still observed in countries with high vaccine coverage. New vaccination schemes against pertussis have been developed to reduce the risk of serious illness in young infants and young children. It is necessary that all children worldwide, including HIV-positive individuals, be immunized against pertussis, and every country should seek to reach the entire population with anti-pertussis vaccination and also maintain high coverage (≥90%) at all levels (national and district).

Both the wP and aP vaccines are effective in reducing infant mortality, highlighting the importance of timely vaccination and the need to maintain high coverage, as current data point to a decrease in aP-related immunity. One future challenge may be the improvement of new vaccines considering all these factors, as well as the importance of the production of vaccines against parapertussis, which seems to be more frequent than originally imagined.

Determining the true incidence of pertussis in each country is vital in order for health authorities to devise the best vaccine strategies to control the disease and its consequences.

Author details

Filumena Maria da Silva Gomes*, Maria Helena Valente, Ana Maria de Ulhôa Escobar and Sandra Josefina Ferraz Ellero Grisi

*Address all correspondence to: filumena.gomes@fm.usp.br

Department of Pediatrics, Faculdade de Medicina FMUSP, Universidade de São Paulo, São Paulo, SP, Brazil

References

[1] Cherry JD, Heininger U. Pertussis and other *Bordetella*. In: Cherry JD, Demmler-Harrison GJ, Kaplan SL, Hotez P, Steinbach WJ, editors. Feigin & Cherry's Textbook of Pediatric Infectious Diseases. 7th ed. Philadelphia, PA: Elsevier-Sauders; 2014. pp. 1616-1639

[2] Nadel S. Infectious Diseases in the Pediatric Intensive Care Unit. London: Springer; 2008

[3] WHO 2014. WHO SAGE pertussis working group Background paper SAGE April 2014. Available: http://www.who.int/immunization/sage/meetings/2014/april/1_Pertussis_background_FINAL4_web.pdf [Accessed: 18 Oct 2017]

[4] Provisional Pertussis Surveillance Report. CDC 2017. Morbidity and Mortality Weekly Report. 2017;**65**(52):1496. Available: https://www.cdc.gov/pertussis/downloads/pertuss-surv-report-2016-provisional.pdf [Accessed: 01 Nov 2017]

[5] Dalby T, Andersen PH, Hoffmann S. Epidemiology of pertussis in Denmark, 1995 to 2013. Euro Surveillance. 2016;**21**(36):1-8

[6] Nieves DJ, Heininger U. Bordetella pertussis. Microbiology Spectrum. 2016;**4**(3):EI10-0008-2015

[7] Souder E, Long SS. Pertussis in the era of new strains of *Bordetella pertussis*. Infectious Disease Clinics of North America. 2015;**29**:699-713

[8] Pittet LF, Emonet S, François P, Bonetti E-J, Schrenzel J, Hug M, et al. Diagnosis of whooping cough in Switzerland: Differentiating Bordetella pertussis from Bordetella holmesii by polymerase chain reaction. PLoS One. 2014;**9**(2):e88936

[9] Centers for Disease Control and Prevention (CDC). Updated Recommendations for Use of Tetanus Toxoid, Reduced Diphtheria Toxoid and Acellular Pertussis Vaccine (Tdap) in Pregnant Women and Persons Who Have or Anticipate Having Close Contact with an Infant Aged <12 Months—Advisory Committee on Immunization Practices (ACIP) 2011. Morbidity and Mortality Weekly Report. 2011;**60**(41):1424-1426

[10] Bento AI, King AA, Rohani P. Maternal pertussis immunisation: Clinical gains and epidemiological legacy. Euro Surveillance. 2017:**22**(15):pii. 30510

[11] Gaillard ME, Bottero D, Moreno G, Rumbo M, Hozbor D. Strategies and new developments to control pertussis, an actual health problem. Pathogens and Disease. 2015; **73**(8):ftv059

[12] Winter K, Nickell S, Powell M, Harriman K. Effectiveness of prenatal versus postpartum tetanus, diphtheria, and acellular pertussis vaccination in preventing infant pertussis. Clinical Infectious Diseases. 2017;**64**(1):3-8

[13] Winter K, Nickell S, Powell M, Harriman K. Effectiveness of prenatal versus postpartum tetanus, diphtheria, and acellular pertussis vaccination on pertussis severity in infants. Clinical Infectious Diseases. 2017;**64**(1):9-14

[14] McGirr A, Fisman DN. Duration of pertussis immunity after DtaP immunization: A meta-analysis. Pediatrics. 2015;**135**:331-343

[15] Wright SW, Edwards KM, Decker M, Zeldin MH. Pertussis infection in adults with persistent cough. Journal of the American Medical Association. 1995;**273**:1044-1046

[16] WHO. Pertussis vaccines: WHO position paper, August 2015 – Recommendations. Vaccine. 2016;**34**:1423-1425

[17] Cherry JD. Pertussis: Challenges today and for the future. PLoS Pathogens. 2013;**9**(7): e1003418

[18] ECDC 2016. European Centre for Disease Prevention and Control. Annual Epidemiological Report 2016—Pertussis. Stockholm: ECDC; 2016. Available from: http://ecdc.europa.eu/en/healthtopics/Pertussis/Pages/Annualepidemiologicalreport2016.aspx [Accessed: 25 Oct 2017]

[19] Gkentzi D, Katsakiori P, Marangos M, Hsia Y, Amirthalingam G, Heath PT, Ladhani S. Maternal vaccination against pertussis: A systematic review of the recent literature. Archives of Disease in Childhood. Fetal and Neonatal Edition. 2017;**102**(5):F456-F463

[20] Esposito S, Principi N, for the European Society of Clinical Microbiology and Infectious Diseases (ESCMID) Vaccine Study Group (EVASG). Immunization against pertussis in adolescents and adults. Clinical Microbiology and Infection. 2016;**22**(Suppl 5):S89-S95

[21] WHO 2017. WHO Global Health Observatory data repository. Pertussis. Reported cases by WHO region: 2017-07-17. Available: http://apps.who.int/gho/data/view.main.1520_43?lang=en [Accessed: 01 Nov 2017]

[22] Matthias J, Pritchard PS, Martin SW, Dusek C, Cathey E, D'Alessio R, et al. Sustained transmission of pertussis in vaccinated, 1-5-year-old children in a preschool, Florida, USA. Emerging Infectious Diseases. 2016;**22**(2):242-246

[23] Bart MJ, Harris SR, Advani A, Arakawa Y, Bottero D, Cassiday PK, et al. Global population structure and evolution of *Bordetella pertussis* and their relationship with vaccination. MBio. 2014;**5**(2):e01074-e01014

[24] Van Gent M, Heuvelman CJ, van der Heide HG, Hallander HO, Advani A, Guiso N, et al. Analysis of *Bordetella pertussis* clinical isolates circulating in European countries during the period 1998-2012. European Journal of Clinical Microbiology & Infectious Diseases. 2015;**34**(4):821-830

[25] Martini H, Rodeghiero C, van den Poel C, Vincent M, Pierard D, Huygen K. Pertussis diagnosis in Belgium: Results of the National Reference Centre for Bordetella anno 2015. Epidemiology and Infection. 2017;**145**(11):2366-2373

[26] Breakwell L, Kelso P, Finley C, Schoenfeld S, Goode B, Misegades LK, et al. Pertussis vaccine effectiveness in the setting of pertactin-deficient pertussis. Pediatrics. 2016;**137**(5):pii: e20153973

[27] Bailon H, León-Janampa N, Hozbor D. Increase in pertussis cases along with high prevalence of two emerging genotypes of Bordetella pertussis in Perú, 2012. BMC Infectious Diseases. 2016;**16**:422

[28] CDC 2017. NNDSS (National Notifiable Diseases Surveillance System) Surveillance Case Definitions/Pertussis: Pertussis/Whooping Cough (*Bordetella pertussis*) 2014 Case Definition. Available: https://wwwn.cdc.gov/nndss/conditions/pertussis/case-definition/2014/ [Accessed: 01 Nov 2017]

[29] CDC 2017. CDC/Pertussis Home /Pertussis in Other Countries/Latin American Pertussis Project/Countries/Brazil/Pertussis in Brazil Brazil's Epidemiologic Bulletins, and Tables of Reported Cases and Deaths due to Pertussis. Available: https://www.cdc.gov/pertussis/countries/lapp-brazil.html [Accessed: 01 Nov 2017]

[30] Navarro-Alonso JA, Taboada-Rodríguez JA, Limia-Sánchez A. Nuevo calendário de Vacunación para Espana, 2016 (parte 2). Revista Española de Salud Pública. 2016;**90**:e1-e9

[31] Sala-Farré M-R, Arias-Varela C, Recasens-Recasens A, Simó-Sanahuja, Munoz-Almagro C, Pérez-Jové J. Pertussis epidemic despite high levels of vaccination coverage with acellular pertussis vaccine. Enfermedades Infecciosas y Microbiología Clínica. 2015;**33**(1):27-31

[32] Solano R, Masa-Calles J, Garib Z, Grullón P, Santiago SL, Brache A, Domínguez A, Cayla JA. Epidemiology of pertussis in two Ibero-American countries with different vaccination policies: Lessons derived from different surveillance systems. BMC Public Health. 2016;**16**:1178

[33] Duterme S, Vanhoof R, Vansderpas J, Pierard D, Huygen K. Serodiagnosis of whooping cough in Belgium: Results of the National Reference Centre for *Bordetella pertussis* anno 2013. Acta Clinica Belgica. 2016;**71**(2):86-91

[34] Heininger U, André P, Chlibek R, Kristufkova Z, Kutsar K, Mangarov A, et al. Comparative epidemiologic characteristics of pertussis in 10 central and eastern European countries, 2000-2013. PLoS One. 2016;**11**(6):e0155949

[35] Hara M, Fukuoka K, Ozaki I, Ohfuji S, Okada K, Nakano T, et al. Pertussis outbreak in university students and evaluation of acellular pertussis vaccine effectiveness in Japan. BMC Infectious Diseases. 2015;**15**:45

[36] Wanlapakorn N, Ngaovithunvong V, Thongmee T, Vichaiwattana P, Vongpunsawad S, Poovorawan Y. Seroprevalence of antibodies to pertussis toxin among different age groups in Thailand after 37 years of universal whole-cell pertussis vaccination. PLoS One. 2016;**11**(2):e0148338

[37] Clarke C, McIntyre PB, Blyth CC, Wood N, Octavia S, Sintchenko V, et al. The relationship between Bordetella pertussis genotype and clinical severity in Australian children with pertussis. The Journal of Infection. 2016;**72**(2):171-178

[38] Hale S, Quinn HE, Kesson A, Wood NJ, McIntyre PB. Changing patterns of pertussis in a children's hospital in the polymerase chain reaction diagnostic era. The Journal of Pediatrics. 2016;**170**(3):161-165

[39] Celles MD, Magpantay FMG, King AA, Rohani P. The pertussis enigma: Reconciling epidemiology, immunology and evolution. Proceedings of the Royal Society B. 2016; **283**:20152309

[40] Tan T, Dalby T, Forsyth K, Halperin SA, et al. Pertussis across the globe: Recent epidemiologic trends from 2000 to 2013. The Pediatric Infectious Disease Journal. 2015;**34**:e222-e232

[41] Meeting of the Strategic Advisory Group of Experts on immunization. April 2017–Conclusions and recommendations. Weekly Epidemiological Record. 2017;**92**(22):301-320

[42] Rocha G, Soares P, Soares H, Pissara S, Guimarães H. Pertussis in the newborn: Certainties and uncertainties in 2014. Paediatric Respiratory Reviews. 2015;**16**(2):112-118

[43] CDC 2017. CDC Vaccines & Preventable Diseases Home Vaccines by Disease Diphtheria, Tetanus, and Whooping Cough Vaccination: What Everyone Should Know Available: https://www.cdc.gov/vaccines/vpd/dtap-tdap-td/public/index.html [Accessed: 03 Nov 2017]

[44] Sigera S, Perera J, Rasarathinam J, Samaranayake D, Ediriweera D. Seroprevalence of Bordetella pertussis specific immunoglobulin G antibody levels among asymptomatic individuals aged 4 to 24 years: A descriptive cross sectional study from Sri Lanka. BMC Infectious Diseases. 2016 Dec 1;**16**(1):729

[45] Williams WW, Lu PJ, O'Halloran A, Bridges CB, Pilishvili T, Hales CM, Markowitz LE, Centers for Disease Control and Prevention (CDC). Noninfluenza vaccination coverage among adults—United States, 2012. Morbidity and Mortality Weekly Report. 2014;**63**(5): 95-102

[46] Curtis CR, Baughman AL, DeBolt C, Goodykoontz S, Kenyon C, et al. Risk factors associated with Bordetella pertussis among infants aged <4 months in the pre-Tdap era—United States, 2002-2005. The Pediatric Infectious Diseases Journal. 2017;**36**(8):726-735

[47] Forsyth K, Plotkin S, Tan T, Konig W. Strategies to decrease pertussis transmission to infants. Pediatrics. 2015;**135**(6):e1475-e1482

[48] Sukumaran L, McCarthy NL, Kharbanda EO, McNeil MM, Nafeway AL, et al. Association of Tdap vaccination with acute events and adverse birth outcomes among pregnant women with prior tetanus-containing immunizations. Journal of the American Medical Association. 2015;**314**(15):1581-1587

[49] Winter K, Cherry JD, Harriman L. Effectiveness of prenatal tetanus, diphtheria, and acellular pertussis vaccination on pertussis severity in infants. Clinical Infectious Diseases. 2017;**64**(1):9-14

[50] Kharbanda EO, Vazquez-Benitez G, Lipkind HS, Klein NP, Cheetham C, et al. Evaluation of the association of maternal pertussis vaccination with obstetric events and birth outcomes. Journal of the American Medical Association. 2014;**312**(18):1897-1904

[51] CDC. CDC. Updated recommendations for use of tetanus toxoid, reduced diphtheria toxoid, and acellular pertussis vaccine (Tdap) in pregnant women–advisory committee on immunization practices (ACIP), 2012. Morbidity and Mortality Weekly Report. 2013;**62**(07):131-135

[52] Berenson AB, Hirth JM, Rahman M, Laz YH, Rupp RE, Sarpong KO. Maternal and infant outcomes among women vaccinated against pertussis during pregnangy. Human Vaccines & Immunotherapeutics. 2016;**12**(8):1965-1971

[53] Van Savage J, Decker MD, Edwards KM, Sell SH, Karzon DT. Natural history of pertussis antibody in the infant and effect on vaccine response. The Journal of Infectious Diseases. 1990;**161**:487-492

[54] Eberhardt CS, Blanchard-Rohner G, Lemaitre B, Boukrid M, Combescure C, Othenin-Girard V, et al. Maternal Immunization earlier in pregnancy maximizes antibody transfer and expected infant seropositivity against pertussis. Clinical Infectious Diseases. 2016;**62**(7):829-836

[55] Raya BA, Srugo I, Kessel A, Peterman M, Vaknin A, Bamberger E. The decline of pertussis-specific antibodies after tetanus, diphtheria, and acellular pertussis immunization in late pregnancy. The Journal of Infectious Diseases. 2015;**212**(12):1869-1873

[56] Niewiesk S. Maternal antibodies: Clinical significance, mechanism of interference with immune responses, and possible vaccination strategies. Frontiers in Immunology. 2014;**5**:446

[57] Ladhani SN, Andrews NJ, Southern J, Jones CE, Amirthalingam G, Waight PA, et al. Antibody responses after primary immunization in infants born to women receiving a pertussis-containing vaccine during pregnancy: Single arm observational study with a historical comparator. Clinical Infectious Diseases. 2015;**61**:1637-1644

[58] Maertens K, Caboré RN, Huygen K, Vermeiren S, Hens N, et al. Pertussis vaccination during pregnancy in Belgium: Follow-up of infants until 1 month after the fourth infant pertussis vaccination at 15 months of age. Vaccine. 2016;**34**:3613-3619

[59] Maertens K, Caboré RN, Huygen K, Hens N, Van Damme P, Leuridan E. Pertussis vaccination during pregnancy in Belgium: Results of a prospective controlled cohort study. Vaccine. 2016;**34**:142-150

[60] Carcione D, Regan AK, Tracey L, Mak DB, Gibbs R, Dowse GK, et al. The impact of parental postpartum pertussis vaccination on infection in infants: A population-based study of cocooning in Western Australia. Vaccine. 2015;**33**:5654-5661

[61] Baxter R, Bartlett J, Fireman B, Lewis E, Klein NP. Effectiveness of vaccination during pregnancy to prevent infant pertussis. Pediatrics. 2017;**139**(5):e20164091

[62] Walther K, Burckhardt M-A, Erb T, Heininger U. Implementation of pertussis immunization in health-care personnel. Vaccine. 2015;**33**:2009-2014

Section 3

Current Pertussis Vaccines and Strategies

Chapter 4

Preventive and Protective Properties of Pertussis Vaccines: Current Situation and Future Challenges

De-Simone SG, Provance DW and Rocha da Silva F

Additional information is available at the end of the chapter

http://dx.doi.org/10.5772/intechopen.75055

Abstract

Pertussis, more commonly known as whooping cough, is a potentially fatal respiratory disease caused by *Bordetella pertussis*. Two different types of vaccines provide effective protection: killed whole-cell vaccines (wPV) and more recently available acellular vaccines (aPVs) formulated with specific components. Disturbingly, while the vaccines are widely used, the incidence of disease is increasing in several developed countries that have switched from wPV to an aPV. It is suggested that the single most important underlying cause suggested for the resurgence is transmission through asymptomatic infections. While both vaccines protect against disease, a newly developed baboon model has shown that they do not prevent infection. Importantly, wPV-vaccinated animals appeared to clear an infection more rapidly than those vaccinated with aPV, which can relate to the period of possible disease transmission. To ultimately control whooping cough, it is clear that a more effective vaccine is needed that can prevent both disease and transmission. Modifications underway include the elimination of LPS from wPVs to improve their safety profiles and augmentation of aPVs with other bacterium proteins to increase immunogenicity and the longevity of protection. In the interim, vaccinations with aPV during pregnancy appear to protect newborns, the most susceptible to deadly pertussis.

Keywords: pertussis, whooping cough, whole-cell vaccine, acellular vaccine, herd protection

1. Introduction

Pertussis or whooping cough, caused by *Bordetella pertussis*, is a severe respiratory childhood disease that can be fatal, particularly in very young infants. However, it also represents a significant disease burden in older children, adolescents, and adults [1]. The first pertussis vaccine was developed in 1926 [2] but has only been available for large-scale administration

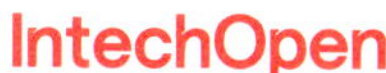

since the middle of the last century. Today, more efficacious vaccines based on key antigens of pertussis have been developed and are available for providing global coverage in vaccination programs [3]. These vaccines are included on the World Health Organization (WHO) Model List of Essential Medicines, as one of the most effective and safe medicines needed in a healthcare system [4]. Nevertheless, the disease is still not under control and today is considered one of the most prevalent vaccine-preventable childhood diseases. The World Health Organization (WHO) records close to 160,700 pertussis-related deaths in children younger than 5 years in 2014 and more than 24.1 million yearly pertussis cases worldwide [5]. Since the 1950s, the incidence and the numbers of pertussis-linked deaths have declined dramatically and reached its lowest point in several countries in the late 1970s, which showed the effectiveness of mass vaccination programs against pertussis. Prior to their implementation, the reported incidence of the disease was as high as 150 cases per 100,000 persons, which was most likely a vast underestimation even in countries like the USA [6]. More recently, the number of cases and associated deaths has again increased in several industrialized countries, reflecting a shortcoming in current vaccination strategies.

Two types of pertussis vaccines (PVs) are currently available: the first-generation whole-cell vaccines (wPV) and the more recent acellular vaccines (aPVs). While the efficacy of wPV (**Table 1**) has been demonstrated to be ≥94% after three administrations [7], the occurrence of adverse local and systemic events along with difficulties in production consistency leads to the development of aPVs in the 1980s, currently composed of one to five purified key antigens (**Table 2**). All available aPVs are combined with tetanus and diphtheria toxoids. Several are also formulated with hepatitis B, inactivated polio, and *Haemophilus influenza* B polysaccharide [8]. The aPVs clearly have an improved safety profile over wPV, and their short-term efficacy after three administrations was estimated to be 67–70% up to 84%, even those containing three or five *B. pertussis* components [8]. This value was recently confirmed in a systematic review of meta-analysis data focusing on the short-term protective effect of currently available childhood pertussis vaccines [9]. Because of their improved safety profiles and similar efficacies, most

Manufacturer or Distributor	Country
Behringwerke	Germany
CSL Limited	Australia
Institute of Technology in Immunobiology (Bio-Manguinhos) / Butantan Institut	Brazil
Merck Sharp @ Dohme	USA
Pasteur/Mérieux	France
SmithKline Beecham	USA
Wyeth-LederleVaccines and Pediatrics (Wyeth-Ayerst Laboratories)	Germany/Austria

Table 1. List of whole cell pertussis vaccine manufacturers or distributors.

Name of aPVs	Composition[1]	Manufacturers/Distributer
[2]Acel-Imune	(PT, FHA, PRN, FIM) +DT+TT	Wyeth Pharmaceutics (USA)
[2]Acelluvax (Triacelluvax)	(PT, FHA, PRN) +DT+TT	Chiron Vaccines (USA)
[3]Adacel	(PT, FHA, PRN, FIM) +DT+TT	Sanofi Pasteur
[4]Boostrix-3	(PT, FHA, PRN) +DT+TT	Sanofi Pasteur
BSc-1	(PT)	Biocine Sclavo
CLL-3F2	(PT, FHA, FIM)	Sanofi Pasteur (Canada)
Certiva	(PT)+DT+TT	Baxter Laboratory
Daptacel (Tripacel)	(PT, FHA, PRN, FIM) +DT+TT	Sanofi Pasteur
[5]DTaP-HB-IPV-Hib	PT, FHA, PRN, FIM) +DT+TT + HB + IPV + Hib	MGM Vacines Co (Merck/Sanofi)
[6]2HCPDT	(PT, FHA, PRN, FIM) +DT+TT	Sanofi Pasteur (Canada)
Infanrix	(PT, FHA, PRN) + DT+TT	Glaxo Smith Klein (Rixensant, Belgium)
[7]JNIM-7	(PT)	Japan Nat Inst of Healthy
LPB-3P	(PT, FHA, PRN)	Wyeth Lederle Vaccines and Pediatric (Germany)
MIch-2	(PT, FHA)	Michigan Department of Public Health
[8]NIH-6	(PT, FHA)	Japan Nat Inst of Healthy
[9]Pentavac	(PT, FHA, PRN, FIM) +DT+TT + HB + IPV + Hib	Sanofi Pasteur (France)
Por-3F2	(PT, FHA, FIM)	Speywood (Porton) Pharmaceuticals
[10]Repevax	(PT, FHA, PRN, FIM) +DT+TT + IPV	Sanofi Pasteur
SSVI-1	(PT)	Swiss Serum and Vaccine Institute
[11]SKB-2	PT, FHA) +DT+TT	SmithKline Beecham Biologicals
Triavax	(PT, FHA) +DT+TT	Sanofi Pasteur (France)
Tripedia	(PT, FHA) +DT+TT	Sanofi Pasteur (USA)

[1]Quantitative difference can be found in the aPV compounds formulations.
[2]No longer available (as of 2013).
[3]A 3-in-1 vaccine, differ from Infanrix by containing reduced quantities of PT (8 μg) + FHA (8 μg) + PRN (2,5 μg) + DT (2.5 lf) + TT (5lf). Licensed for use in person with 4 yr age or older. In the USA 10-60 yr older.
[4] A 3-in-1 vaccine approved for individuals aged ≥10 yr including those aged ≥65 yr.
[5]The 6-in-1 vaccine is given to babies as a series of 3 doses. The first dose is given at 2 months of age, the second at 4 months, and the third at 6 months. The vaccine is given at the same time as other childhood immunizations.
[6]Used in Pentacel and Pediacel.
[7]HCPDT is the "hybrid" formulation of Tripacel, evaluated in 1993 Stockholm trial.
[8]JNIH-6 and 7 were the aPV used in the 1986 Swedish trial.
[9]The 5-in-1 vaccine was used in the UK for many years. In late September 2017 the UK replaced it with a 6-in-1 vaccine for all babies born on or after 1st August 2017. Both vaccines give protection against diphtheria, tetanus, whooping cough (pertussis), polio and Hib disease (*Haemophilus influenzae* type b).
[10]A 3-in1 vaccine indicated for persons from 3 years of age as a booster following primary immunizations.
[11]SKB-2 was an experimental two-company DTaP evaluated in the 1992 Stockholm trial.
Abbreviations: PT, pertussis toxin; FHA, phytohemagglutinin; PRN, pertactin; FIM, fimbriae (mixture of FIM-2 and FIM-3); TT, tetanus toxoid; DT, diphtheria toxoid, HB, Hepatitis B; IPV, Inactived Polio; Hib, *Haemophilus influenzae* type b.

Table 2. Source and composition of acellular pertussis vaccines studied and producers.

developed countries have replaced wPV with an aPV. Globally, wPVs are still the most used vaccines due the higher cost of aPVs, which are difficult to afford in resource-poor countries.

Although the vaccines together have saved millions of people since its introduction, it has been estimated that their effectiveness appears to decrease between 2 and 10% per year [1, 10]. This rate of decrease has been observed in countries that continue to administer wPV. Yet, it has become apparent that the immunity induced by aPV declines substantially faster than that induced by wPV [11, 12], which led the WHO to recommend that countries considering a switch from wPV to aPV should expect further guidance [4]. Multiple studies, both epidemiological and serological, have confirmed that immunity wanes rapidly after the aPV booster at age 4–6 years and the preadolescent dose at age 10–12 years [13–18]. Nonetheless, it appears that the waning immunity induced by aPV, or wPV, is not the only reason for the observed resurgence in pertussis infections.

Another possible mechanism is asymptomatic transmission. Mathematical modeling of the incidence rates of pertussis in the USA and UK supports a role for undetectable transmission in the recent increase cases [19]. The potential for an essentially silent transmission is also supported by observations in a baboon model recently developed for studying *B. pertussis* infections. Vaccinations with aPV did not prevent transmission of *B. pertussis*. Virulent *B. pertussis* continued to establish infections in animals vaccinated with either aPV or wPV, even though both vaccines protected against disease. A major difference observed between the two vaccines was that infections cleared more rapidly in wPV-vaccinated baboons [20]. All vaccinated animals showed a lower total bacterial load compared to naïve animals suggesting that both vaccines have a positive impact to limit the progression of an infection. Yet, it appears that this impact may not be sufficient to control the circulation of *B. pertussis* within a population and could lead to the generation of vaccine escape mutants, which have indeed been observed in several countries where aPV is in use. A likely explanation is the observed increase in the isolation of strains not producing pertactin, due to selective pressure [21]. Conversely, there is no apparent major difference in the pathogenesis of whooping cough in children infected with pertactin-deficient strains compared to pertactin-producing strains. This indicates that pertactin is not required for infection by *B. pertussis* or for the development of the disease, suggesting a role of pertactin in the immune response following vaccination.

In contrast to vaccination with either aPV or wPV, a natural infection by *B. pertussis* is able to induce sterilizing immunity in baboons [20]. This fact is intriguing since studies in human have shown that infection-induced immunity is longer lived than vaccine-induced immunity [22], although probably not lifelong as reinfections have been reported to occur. While the second attacks are very rare, they are usually much milder than the primary infections [23]. Since *B. pertussis* is strictly a mucosal pathogen, it is conceivable that its restricted localization could influence the immunity induced from a natural infection. Although the protective role of mucosal immunity has so far attracted little attention, it may contribute to the differences observed between the protection obtained by a vaccine and a natural infection. These observations suggest that a vaccination approach that more closely mimics a natural infection without resulting in disease may be more successful to ultimately control pertussis.

http://dx.doi.org/10.5772/intechopen.75055

Such a vaccine is currently under development based on a live attenuated *B. pertussis* strain. Named BPZE1, it has been genetically modified to affect the activity of three different toxins such that they are absent, inactive, or minimally active [24]. This strain has been documented to be safe in preclinical models and genetically stable over at least 1 year of continuous passaging in vitro and in vivo in mice [25]. It can induce a strong protection against challenge infections after a single intranasal administration, which lasted at least for up to 1 year. This contrasts with the protection conferred by aPV that can begin to wane after only 6 months. The strain BPZE1 has successfully completed a Phase I clinical trial that showed its safety profile in young male volunteers with a single intranasal dose of up to 10^7 colony-forming units suspended in 100 μl. This trial also showed that BPZE1 can transiently colonize the human nasopharynx and induce *B. pertussis*-specific antibody responses in all colonized individuals. At 6 months, follow-up studies measured antibody titers against all antigens tested to be at least at the same level as detected at 1 month postvaccination. One concern with the trail was the observation that not all subjects showed colonization by BPZE1, even at the highest dose tested, since colonization was found to be essential for the induction of an immune response. A possible reason of the absence of colonization in some individuals may have been their prior contact with wild-type *B. pertussis*, which could have prevented a response to the vaccine. Consistent with this hypothesis is the detection of preexisting antibody titers in the non-colonized individuals that were significantly higher than the pre-vaccination titers of individuals that displayed colonization, especially against pertactin. Additional studies are needed to test the influence of a prior exposure to wild-type *B. pertussis* on BPZE1 colonization and to eliminate the possibility for a previously imperceptible subclinical disease. New clinical trials are in progress to test the hypothesis that the presence of preexisting antibodies prevents colonization by the vaccine strain and to determine if their activity can be neutralized by increasing the vaccine dosage.

Realistically, it would require many more years of research and regulatory approval before a new pertussis vaccine could be available for general use. In the interim, efforts are being made to optimize the application of current vaccines. A promising observation is the protection afforded to newborns, less than 2 months of age, from the immunization of their mothers with aPV during the 28–38th week of gestation. In a recent pertussis outbreak in the UK, the effectiveness of this vaccination schedule was shown to be greater than 90% [26]. Several countries have now made recommendations for providing aPV during pregnancy. However, many issues remain unresolved. For example, the impact of maternal immunization on the immune responses in infants following their primary vaccination is unclear. Several studies have observed a reduction in the primary antibody response to *B. pertussis* antigens following a maternal vaccination [27]. Another issue is the observation that the adoptive caring immunity is effective to prevent disease but does not prevent pertussis infections in neonates [28]. This suggests that the maternal levels of preexisting pertussis-specific antibodies cannot transfer complete protection against infection. The maternal immune system can be activated in response to pertussis and generates a recall response from memory B cells that increases the levels of milk IgA, but the clinical relevance remains to be determined. Lastly, in a mouse model, challenge studies also have shown that antibodies resulting from maternal vaccinations interfere with the functionality of antibodies induced from a subsequent vaccination [29].

2. Resurgence, vaccine design, and new targets

In 2008, there was an estimated incidence of 16 million cases of pertussis infection worldwide that resulted in approximately 195,000 children deaths, making pertussis one of the leading causes of vaccine-preventable deaths in children under 5 years of age [30, 31]. Most of pertussis deaths occur in developing countries. However, pertussis has not only persisted in countries with high vaccination coverage but has resurged with a number of epidemic episodes being recorded [32–34]. The resurgence of pertussis as a deadly childhood disease is a major public health concern that reflects changes in its epidemiology but is also affected by a growing attitude among parents to delay or even refuse vaccination of their children, which highlights the urgent need for new integrated approaches to control the spread and impact of whooping cough. Several explanations have been presented to enlighten the resurgence of pertussis disease over the past few decades in which most of them is associated with the aPVs currently in use: (i) the decrease of vaccine effectiveness over time (declining immunity) [35, 36], (ii) the selection of mutants that can escape the immunity induced by a vaccine [37, 38], and/or (iii) failure of the vaccine to induce sterilizing immunity to the pathogen that avoids transmission [20]. However, perhaps the most significant contributing factor is our relative lack of understanding the basics of pertussis infection, immunity, and disease. We are still unsure of which specific immune responses are protective against *B. pertussis* infection and disease in humans and how to elicit protective responses through vaccination.

To address the resurgence, new vaccination strategies have been explored such as the "cocooning strategy" and maternal immunization. Cocooning refers to the vaccination of mothers and others with direct contact to newborns and infants. Cost-effective cocooning would be difficult to implement since a successful program requires a very high number of contacts be vaccinated to attain a significant impact on the incidence of severe infant pertussis [39]. Currently, there is a growing evidence for effectiveness of immunization of women during pregnancy rather than during the immediate postpartum period. This approach has been found to be more cost-effective than cocooning with a level of vaccine effectiveness against infant deaths that reach an estimated 95% [27]. Alongside the vaccination of contacts, an alternative option under consideration is to advance the vaccination schedule for newborns to 6–8 weeks of age. However, this approach still does not provide protection to infants during their most susceptible period for potentially deadly pertussis infections. A missing element to refinements in the application of available vaccines is an improved surveillance for pertussis. Improvements in the detection of infections and the immune response can positively contribute to evaluations on vaccine efficacy that will help advance our understanding of performance and duration of a pertussis vaccine to provide protection in the field.

Since the 1950s, the toxicity of traditional wPV has been associated with the presence of lipopolysaccharides (LPS), the major constituents of the bacterial outer membranes. To improve on traditional wPVs, the Butantan Institute in Brazil recently produced a wPV with reduced quantities of LPS that removed ≥80% of the endotoxin-related toxicity in comparison to traditional wPV production methods using a chemical extraction of lipo-oligosaccharide (LOS) from the outer membrane. The process maintained the main protective immunogens as well as the integrity of the bacteria in the vaccine [40]. A major challenge over the next few years will be the implementation of a reproducible process that can produce consistent lots under good manufacturing practice conditions.

In recent years, extensive research efforts have elucidated that natural infections and immunizations with wPVs predominantly induce IFN-γ-secreting T-helper 1 cells (Th1) and IL-17-secreting Th17 cells [41–44]. By contrast, it has been shown that aPVs induce a qualitatively different immune response, characterized by the induction of Th2 immunity [39, 43–45]. This difference in the immune response, along with the chemical inactivation of the pertussis toxin antigen in aPVs, may account for the apparent lack of aPV protection against colonization by subsequent *B. pertussis* infections and suboptimal T-cell priming that has been observed as a reduction in the efficiency for the generation of an immune memory repertoire.

Since current aPVs mainly elicit a Th2 response, several solutions have been proposed to improve the Th1/Th17 responses. One possibility is to combine these vaccines with Th1-driving adjuvants, at least for the priming doses [46, 51]. The development of such a candidate vaccine based on a single-immunization platform consisting of three immune stimulators is in progress [47], namely, (i) host defense peptides, (ii) polyphosphazenes (a family of inorganic molecular hybrid polymers based on a phosphorus-nitrogen backbone substituted with organic side groups with very diverse properties), and (iii) the synthetic oligonucleotides containing CpG-ODN (oligodeoxynucleotides) combined with poly(I:C), (polyinosinic-polycytidylic acid) an agonists of Toll-like receptor 9 (TLR9). This last immune stimulatory compound associated with dacarbazine, a therapeutic agent, has been successfully used to promote antitumor immunity [48].

In the case of pertussis, the inclusion of these immune stimulators resulted in a humoral immune response from a single application in neonatal mice and pigs that was 100- to 1000-fold stronger than a licensed aPV [47]. The onset of immunity occurred more quickly with a predominantly Th1 response. Importantly, immunity persisted for more than 2 years and appeared to be highly effective even in the presence of maternal antibodies. To address the contribution of chemically inactivating pertussis toxin to vaccine performance, a strain of *B. pertussis* was engineered as a source for genetically detoxified Ptx for the formulation of a new aPV. In Thai adolescents, its safety was like Adacel, a trivalent aPV combined with diphtheria and tetanus compounds produced by Sanofi Pasteur (see **Table 2)** with an improved induction of neutralizing antibodies against PTx [47].

Substantial evidence has been accumulated in the last 2 years that immunity induced by aPVs is much shorter lived than immunity induced by wPV [10]. Additionally, using refined techniques of peptide microarray, it has been demonstrated that qualitative differences within the humoral response of individuals vaccinated with wPV and aPVs exist. Using a microarray technique, it was shown that animals immunized with wPV recognize qualitatively a major number of B epitopes in the PTx than mice immunized with aPV [49]. Another study using a similar approach compared the recognition pattern of sera from children immunized with different pertussis vaccines (17 *B. pertussis* proteins) and concluded that 11% of the individuals displayed a private humoral response [50]. All these studies are important to guide the rational development of new vaccines.

3. Difficulties with vaccine reformulation

While adults and adolescents normally only experience mild symptoms from a pertussis infection, they are the usual source of infection for neonates, and adoptive maternal immunity does not appear to prevent pertussis in neonates. In a study that compared the specific immune response in mothers of neonates diagnosed with pertussis and mothers of control children [28], preexisting pertussis-specific antibodies were insufficient for protection suggesting that memory B cells play a major role in the adult defense, which is not transferred to neonates. To provide newborns with protection, a new approach would be required, but to change the vaccine given to infants in the first 2 years of life is a discouraging proposition. It would involve a large data set for safety evaluation. Also, the pertussis vaccine is often combined into a multivalent formula with components against other pathogens. Any change directed at improving effectiveness against pertussis would require a recertification process that would impact a wide spectrum of vaccines currently on the market.

More importantly, it would be unethical to conduct formal efficacy studies for new vaccines/formulations that included a non-vaccinated control group. Considering the epidemiological and serological studies that show a rapid decline in immunity after the recommended aPV boosters at ages 4–6 and 10–12 years [13, 15, 16, 18], an intensive focus is being given on the booster vaccines given to preschool-age children and adolescents. However, even for a new booster vaccine, the regulatory pathway is unclear. A classical efficacy study would have to compare a new vaccine with a currently accepted one to show non-inferiority or superiority. Such studies would be expensive and require a long evaluation period considering that the current vaccines are effective for the first couple of years after administration.

Ideally, licensing authorities could present new approaches to evaluate the efficacy of a new vaccine. Alternatives include a greater reliance on the use of protection data obtained from animal studies [52]. The newly developed baboon model could provide in-depth serological data on the levels and duration of antibody titers, which can be verified in smaller human challenge studies using circulating strains of *B. pertussis*. Safety profiles could also be generated from fewer participants if modifications simply involve an update in the components with newer inactivation methods, such as genetic modifications. However, the greatest obstacle is most likely to recruit manufacturers to participate in the development of a new pertussis vaccine or booster. After the tremendous effort and expenditure invested to launch the aPVs along with shifting priorities to new pathogens, major manufacturers are resistant to shouldering multiple and simultaneous clinical development programs [52]. Physicians and government health agencies will be critical to creating a new demand. Assistance from academia and science funding agencies could assist vaccine development by conducting basic research on the pathogenesis and immunology of pertussis along with preliminary clinical trials [52]. All of this implies an enormous effort, but a new pertussis vaccine is needed. It is unethical to continue to allow a vaccine-preventable disease to be incompletely controlled, especially one that prejudices the very young people and disproportionately in less developed countries.

4. Protecting versus vaccination during pregnancy

Since the resurgence of pertussis infection, several studies have shown that the main source of infections in newborns and infants involved close-contact persons, mostly family members [53, 54]. In the first attempt to reduce the incidence of pertussis infections, indirect protection for the reduction of transmission rates was favored, the so-called cocooning strategy. In response, some countries adapted their national immunization guidelines [53–55]. Another study focused on the influence of vaccination rates among siblings and vaccination rates among mothers showed that the provided protection rates are comparable [56, 57]. In contrast, a recent study on the effect of cocooning infants younger than 6 months of age did not detect any reduction in pertussis cases [57]. Besides that, it is not yet clear and has created some controversy if cocoon strategies are cost-effective or even prevent infections [38, 58]. Even in the absence of definitive proof, it is still advisable for recent mothers to know their immunization status as well as those of all potentially close-contact individuals, all of whom can play a critical role in the potential transmission of pertussis to a newborn.

Another means to reduce the rate of pertussis transmission to neonates and young infants is the practice of providing pertussis vaccinations during pregnancy. This has become an important strategy in many countries in the absence of vaccines licensed for use before the age of 6 weeks and unknown effectiveness of cocooning strategies [53, 59–61]. The observation of the transplacental transfer of maternal anti-pertussis antibodies to the fetus led health authorities to first recommend the use of pertussis vaccinations during pregnancy in 2011 [62–64]. In the USA, a maternal vaccination was first recommended after gestational week 20 that was later shifted to a window between weeks 27 and 36 [65]. This recommendation has been adopted by both Switzerland and the UK [64].

Early studies showed that vaccination with Tdap vaccines during gestational week 27–30 + 6 was associated with the highest levels of IgG in umbilical cord blood when compared to vaccination beyond gestational week 31 [59], according to one of the most potent virulence factors of pertussis PTx. A recent study supports these data by showing that the maternal vaccination with Tdap early in the second trimester significantly increased neonatal antibodies at birth in comparison with neonates born from mothers vaccinated in the third trimester [61]. All in all, the antenatal vaccination campaign in the UK achieved a vaccine coverage of 60% with >90% effectiveness [66, 67]. A UK study conducted after initiating maternal vaccinations identified a large reduction in the number of confirmed cases of pertussis infection reported as the cause for a hospital admission that was especially notable for infants younger than 3 months of age [66].

From this campaign, the question arose as to whether a vaccination early in pregnancy might adversely affect the immune response in an infant to vaccinations after birth. Some studies showed that antibody concentrations at birth did not interfere with the immune response to further immunizations after birth [68]. However, it is known that maternally derived antibodies can interfere with the immune response in an infant vaccinated with the same vaccine [68], which was detected after DTaP[1] (administered to children under 7 years of age) vaccination [69]. Maternal antibodies were also shown to interfere with the antibody response to the primary vaccination administered during infancy to children born to Tdap[1] (administered to older children and adults)-vaccinated mothers [62, 70]. Interestingly, a mouse model showed that the vaccination of infant mice reduced the protective functions of maternally derived antibodies in vitro and in vivo [29]. A study that focused on vaccinations with Repevax, a five component aPV combined with tetanus, low-dose diphtheria, and inactivated polio vaccine (Sanofi Pasteur), detected a significant attenuation of pertussis antibodies in infants whose mothers were vaccinated with Repevax during pregnancy [71]. Together with the diminished protection afforded by aPVs, recent findings suggest that the efficacy of current vaccines should be maximized by prenatal vaccination followed by boosting. It is important to continue studies to determine the functionality of maternal antibodies resulting from vaccinations during pregnancy and infant antibodies generated from subsequent vaccinations to better understand the potential for cross interference to design alternative vaccination strategies.

5. Conclusion

It is irrefutable that the worldwide incidence of severe pertussis cases is rising. Nearly 90% of all instances of deaths caused by pertussis occur in infants younger than 4 months of age and are caused by fatal pertussis pneumonia due to PTx activity [72], which highlights the need to inhibit PTx during an acute infection. Over the past few years, the scientific community has responded by initiating studies focused on a better understanding of virulence factors, like PTx, transmission dynamics, and host immune reactions, which can provide a foundation for the generation of a new vaccine but can also guide improvements in the use of current vaccines. It is clear that a control of pertussis requires a durable protection against disease and disruption of transmission. The two types of vaccines available, wPV and aPV, are effective in preventing the disease, but the immunity developed by each wane over time, even more rapidly with aPV, which should encourage countries in which wPV is still in use, not to switch to aPV. Further, transmission from vaccinated individuals is possible since *B. pertussis* can still colonize their respiratory tracts. Improvements to both types are in development, but it will be several years before their widespread use. In the interim, expansions in the use of the current vaccines have been proposed. Cocoon vaccination programs, which are controversial in their effectiveness, rely on generating herd immunity to protect young infants by vaccinating individuals with close contact. In contrast, immunization with aPV during pregnancy can reduce the incidence of severe and deadly pertussis in neonates. However, there are concerns that the antibodies raised from the maternal immunization can interfere with the immune response in the child to their primary vaccination. All approaches under development would benefit from

---

[1]DTaP, Tdap, and Td are all similar vaccines, given for the same diseases at different times of life. Depending on the age, certain amounts of vaccine components are administered. Typing uppercase and lowercase letters denotes the component of the vaccine and the quantities in it. Uppercase letters in abbreviations denote undiluted doses of diphtheria (D), tetanus (T), and pertussis (P) toxoids. The lowercase letters d and p denote reduced doses of diphtheria and pertussis toxoids used in formulations for adolescents and adults. The letter a in the DTaP and Tdap vaccines means acellular.

a more detailed surveillance program to determine the rates of symptomatic and asymptomatic infections as well as an examination of the genetic diversity of *B. pertussis* strains in circulation to better understand methods to prevent the impacts of infection.

Acknowledgements

SGS received support from the Brazilian Council for Scientific Research (CNPq-n° 467.488.2014-2), Carlos Chagas Filho Foundation for Research Support of Rio de Janeiro State (FAPERJ n° E-26 110.198-13), and Higher Education Coordination for the Improvement (CAPES-n° 2919-2010).

Conflict of interest

The authors declare no conflict of interest.

Author details

De-Simone SG[1,2,3]*, Provance DW[1] and Rocha da Silva F[2]

*Address all correspondence to: dsimone@cdts.fiocruz.br

1 FIOCRUZ, Center for Technological Development in Health (CDTS)/National Institute of Science and Technology for Innovation in Neglected Diseases (INCT-IDN), Rio de Janeiro, RJ, Brazil

2 FIOCRUZ, Oswaldo Cruz Institute, Laboratory of Experimental and Computational Biochemistry of Pharmaceuticals, Rio de Janeiro, RJ, Brazil

3 Molecular and Cellular Biology Department, Biology Institute, Federal Fluminense University, Niterói, RJ, Brazil

References

[1] Hewlett EL, Edwards KM. Clinical practice. Pertussis-not just for kids. The New England Journal of Medicine. 2005;**352**:1215-1222. DOI: 10.1056/NEJMcp041025

[2] Macera CA, Shaffer R, Shaffer PM. Introduction to Epidemiology: Distribution and Determinants of Disease in Humans. 1st ed. Boston, MA, USA: Cengage Learning; 2013. p 251

[3] de Gouw D, Diavatopoulos DA, Bootsma HJ, Hermans PW, Mooi FR. Pertussis: A matter of immune modulation. FEMS Microbiology Reviews. 2011;**35**:441-474. DOI: 10.1111/j.1574-6976.2010.00257.x

[4] WHO. Meeting of the strategic advisory group of experts on immunization, April 2014—Conclusions and recommendations. Weekly Epidemiological Record. 2014;**89**:221-236

[5] Yeung KHT, Duclos P, Nelson EAS, Hutubessy RCW. An update of the global burden of pertussis in children younger than 5 years: A modelling study. The Lancet Infectious Diseases. 2017;**17**:974-980. DOI: 10.1016/S1473-3099(17)30390-0

[6] Mooi FR, van Loo IH, van Gent M, He Q, Bart MJ, Heuvelman KJ, et al. *Bordetella pertussis* strains with increased toxin production associated with pertussis resurgence. Emerging Infectious Diseases. 2009;**15**:1206-12213. DOI: 10.3201/eid1508.08151

[7] Guiso N, Hegerle N. Other Bordetellas, lessons for and from pertussis vaccines. Expert Review of Vaccines. 2014;**13**:1125-1133. DOI: 10.1586/14760584.2014.942221

[8] SmithKline Beecham Biologicals. Synopsis of Final Study Report 217744/025 (DTPa-HBV-IPV-025); 1999

[9] Fulton TR, Phadke VK, Orenstein WA, Hinman AR, Johnson WD, et al. Protective effect of contemporary Pertussis vaccines: A systematic review and meta-analysis. Clinical Infectitious Diseases. 2016;**62**:100-110. DOI: 10.1093/cid/ciw051

[10] Koepke R, Eickhoff JC, Ayele RA, Petit AB, Schauer SL, et al. Estimating the effectiveness of tetanus-diphtheria-acellular pertussis vaccine (TDaP) for preventing pertussis: Evidence of rapidly waning immunity and difference in effectiveness by TDaP brand. The Journal of Infectious Diseases. 2014;**210**:942-953. DOI: 10.1093/infdis/jiu322

[11] Witt MA, Katz PH, Witt DJ. Unexpectedly limited durability of immunity following acellular pertussis vaccination n preadolescents in a North American outbreak. Clinical Infectious Diseases. 2012;**54**:1730-1735. DOI: 10.1093/cid/cis287

[12] Gambhir M, Clark TA, Cauchemez S, Tartof SY, Swerdlow DL, et al. A change in vaccine efficacy and duration of protection explains recent rises in pertussis incidence in the United States. PLoS Computational Biology. 2015;**11**:e1004138. DOI: 10.1371/journal.pcbi.1004138

[13] Misegades LK, Winter K, Harriman K, Talarico J, Messonnier NE, et al. Association of childhood pertussis with receipt of 5 doses of pertussis vaccine by time since last vaccine dose, California, 2010. JAMA. 2012;**308**:2126-2132. DOI: 10.1001/jama.2012.14939

[14] Sheridan SL, Ware RS, Grimwood K, Lambert SB. Number and order of whole cell pertussis vaccines in infancy and disease protection. JAMA. 2012;**308**:454-456. DOI: 10.1001/jama.2012.6364

[15] Baxter R, Bartlett J, Rowhani-Rahbar A, Fireman B, Klein NP. Effectiveness of pertussis vaccines for adolescents and adults: Case-control study. BMJ. 2013;**347**:f4249. DOI: 10.1136/bmj.f4249

[16] Klein NP, Bartlett J, Fireman B, Rowhani-Rahbar A, Baxter R. Comparative effectiveness of acellular versus whole-cell pertussis vaccines in teenagers. Pediatrics. 2013;**131**:e1716-e1722. DOI: 10.1542/peds.2012-3836

[17] Liko J, Robison SG, Cieslak PR. Priming with whole-cell versus acellular pertussis vaccine. The New England Journal of Medicine. 2013;**368**:581-582. DOI: 10.1056/NEJMc1212006

[18] Tartof SY, Lewis M, Kenyon C, White K, Osborn A, et al. Waning immunity to pertussis following 5 doses of DTaP. Pediatrics. 2013;**131**:e1047-e1052. DOI: 10.1542/peds.2012-1928

[19] Althouse BM, Scarpino SV. Asymptomatic transmission and the resurgence of *Bordetella pertussis*. BMC Medicine. 2015;**13**:146. DOI: 10.1186/s12916-015-0382-8

[20] Warfel JM, Zimmerman LI, Merkel TJ. Acellular pertussis vaccines protect against disease but fail to prevent infection and transmission in a nonhuman primate model. PNAS. 2014; **111**:787-792. DOI: 10.1073/pnas.1314688110

[21] Martin SW, Pawloski L, Williams M, Weening K, DeBolt C, Qin X, et al. Pertactin negative *Bordetella pertussis* strains: Evidence for a possible selective advantage. Clinical Infectious Diseases. 2015;**60**:223-227. DOI: 10.1093/cid/ciu788

[22] Le Coustumier A, Njamkepo E, Cattoir V, Guillot S, Guiso N. *Bordetella petrii* infection with long-lasting persistence in human. Emerging Infectious Diseases. 2011;**17**:612-618. DOI: 10.3201/eid1704.101480

[23] Cherry JD, Grimprel E, Guiso N, Heininger U, Mertsola J. Defining pertussis epidemiology: Clinical, microbiologic and serologic perspectives. The Pediatric Infectious Disease Journal. 2005;**24**:S25-S34. DOI: 10.1097/01.inf.0000160926.89577.3b

[24] Kliegman R, Stanton B, St Geme J, Schor N, editors. Textbook of Pediatrics. 20th ed. Philadelphia: Elsevier; 2015; 197p

[25] Thorstensson R, Trollfors B, Al-Tawil N, Jahnmatz M, Bergström J, Ljungman M, et al. A Phase I clinical study of a live attenuated Bordetella pertussis vaccine—BPZE1; a single centre, double-blind, placebo-controlled, dose escalating study of bpze1 given intranasally to healthy adult male volunteers. PLoS One;**9**:e83449. DOI: 10.1371/journal.pone.0083449

[26] Amirthalingam G, Campbel H, Ribeiro S, Fry NK, Ramsay M, Miller E, Andrews N. Sustained effectiveness of the maternal pertussis immunization program in England 3 years. Clinical Infectitious Diseases. 2016;**63**:S236-S243. DOI: 10.1093/cid/ciw559

[27] Chiappini E, Stival A, Galli L, de Martino M. Pertussis re-emergence in the post-vaccination era. BMC Infectious Diseases. 2013;**26, 13**:151. DOI: 10.1186/1471-2334-13-151

[28] Marcellini V, Piano-Mortari E, Fedele G, Gesualdo F, Pandolfi E, et al. Protection against Pertussis in humans correlates to elevated serum antibodies and memory B cells. Frontiers in Immunology. 2017;**8**:1158. DOI: 10.3389/fimmu.2017.01158

[29] Feunou PF, Mielcareck N, Locht C. Reciprocal interference of maternal and infant immunization in protection against pertussis. Vaccine. 2016;**34**:1062-1969. DOI: 10.1016/j.vaccine.2016.01.011

[30] Black RE, Cousens S, Johnson HL, Lawn JE, Rudan I, et al. Global, regional, and national causes of child mortality in 2008: A systematic analysis. Lancet. 2010;**375**:1969. DOI: 10.1016/S0140-6736(10)60549-1

[31] Gall SA. Prevention of pertussis, tetanus, and diphtheria among pregnant, postpartum women, and infants. Clinical Obstetrics and Gynecology. 2012;**55**:498-509. DOI: 10.1097/GRF.0b013e.31824f3b38

[32] Cherry JD. Epidemic pertussis in 2012—The resurgence of a vaccine-preventable disease. The New England Journal of Medicine. 2012;**367**:785. DOI: 10.1056/NEJMp1209051

[33] Winter K, Glaser C, Watt J, Harriman K. Centers for Disease Control and Prevention (CDC). Pertussis epidemic–California. MMWR. Morbidity and Mortality Weekly Report. 2014;**63**:1129-1132

[34] Tan T, Dalby T, Forsyth K, Halperin SA, Heininger U, et al. Pertussis across the globe: Recent epidemiologic trends from 2000-2013. The Pediatric Infectious Disease Journal. 2015;**34**:e222-ee32. DOI: 10.1097/INF.0000000000000795

[35] Wendelboe AM, Van Rie A, Salmaso S, Englund JA. Duration of immunity against pertussis after natural infection or vaccination. The Pediatric Infectious Disease Journal. 2005;**4**:S58-S61. DOI: 10.1097/01.inf.0000160914.59160.41

[36] McGirr A, Fisman DN. Duration of pertussis immunity after DTaP immunization: A meta-analysis. Pediatrics. 2015;**135**:331-343. DOI: 10.1542/peds.2014-1729

[37] Mooi FR, van Loo IH, King AJ. Adaptation of *Bordetella pertussis* to vaccination: A cause for its reemergence? Emerging Infectious Diseases. 2001;**7**:526-528. DOI: 10.3201/eid0707.010708

[38] Bart MJ, Harris SR, Advani A, Arakawa Y, Bottero D, et al. Global population structure and evolution of *Bordetella pertussis* and their relationship with vaccination. mBio. 2014;**5**:e01074. DOI: 10.1128/mBio.01074-14

[39] Swamy GK, Wheeler SM. Neonatal pertussis, cocooning and maternal immunization. Expert Review of Vaccines. 2014;**13**:1107-1114. DOI: 10.1586/14760584.2014.944509

[40] Dias WO, van der Ark AAJ, Sakaushi MA, Kubrusly FS, Prestes AFRO, et al. An improved whole cell pertussis with reduced content of endotoxin. Human Vaccines & Immunotherapeutics. 2013;**9**:339-348. DOI: 10.4161/hv.22847

[41] Rieber N, Graf A, Belohradsky BH, Hartl D, Urschel S, et al. Differences of humoral and cellular immune response to an acellular pertussis booster in adolescents with a whole cell or acellular primary vaccination. Vaccine. 2008;**26**:6929-6235. DOI: 10.1016/j.vaccine.2008.09.064

[42] Fedele G, Spensieri F, Palazzo R, Nasso M, Cheung GY, et al. *Bordetella pertussis* commits human dendritic cells to promote a Th1/Th17 response through the activity of adenylate cyclase toxin and MAPK-pathways. PLoS One. 2010;**5**:e8734. DOI: 10.1371/journal.pone.0008734

[43] Ross PJ, Sutton CE, Higgins S, Allen AC, Walsh K, Misiak A, Lavelle EC, McLoughlin RM, Mills KH. Relative contribution of Th1 and Th17 cells in adaptive immunity to *Bordetella*

pertussis: Towards the rational design of an improved acellular pertussis vaccine. PLoS Pathogens. 2013;**9**:e1003264. DOI: 10.1371/journal.ppat.1003264

[44] Warfel JM, Merkel TJ. *Bordetella pertussis* infection induces a mucosal IL-17 response and long-lived Th17 and Th1 immune memory cells in nonhuman primates. Mucosal Immunology. 2013;**6**:787-796. DOI: 10.1038/mi.2012.117

[45] Ausiello CM, Lande R, Urbani F, Di Carlo B, Stefanelli P, et al. Cell-mediated immunity and antibody responses to *Bordetella pertussis* antigens in children with a history of pertussis infection and in recipients of an acellular pertussis vaccine. The Journal of Infectitious Diseases. 2000;**181**:1989-1995. DOI: 10.1086/315509

[46] Allen AC, Mills KH. Improved pertussis vaccines based on adjuvants that induce cell-mediated immunity. Expert Review of Vaccines. 2014;**13**:1253-1264. DOI: 10.1586/14760584.2014.936391

[47] Carbonetti NH, von König CHW, Lan R, Jacob-Dubuisson F, Cotter PA, et al. Highlights of the 11th International Bordetella symposium: From basic biology to vaccine development. Clinical and Vaccine Immunology. 2016;**23**:842-850. DOI: 10.1128/IAI.01578-06

[48] Noci V, Tortoreto M, Gulino A, Storti C, Bianchi F, Zaffaroni N, Tripodo C, Tagliabue E, Balsari A, Sfondrini L. Poly(I:C) and CpG-ODN combined aerosolization to treat lung metastases and counter the immunosuppressive microenvironment. Oncoimmunology. 2015;**4**:e1040214. DOI: 10.1080/2162402X.2015.1040214

[49] Silva FR, Napoleão-Pego P, De-Simone SG. Identification of linear B epitopes of pertactin of *Bordetella pertussis* induced by immunization with whole and acellular vaccine. Vaccine. 2014;**32**:6251-6258. DOI: 10.1016/j.vaccine.2014.09.019

[50] Valentini D, Ferrara G, Advani R, Hallander HO, Maeurer MJ. Serum reactome induced by *Bordetella pertussis* infection and Pertussis vaccines: Qualitative differences in serum antibody recognition patterns revealed by peptide microarray analysis. BMC Immunology. 2015;**16**:40. DOI: 10.1186/s12865-015-0090-3

[51] Locht C. Pertussis: Acellular, whole-cell, new vaccines, what to choose? Expert Review of Vaccines. 2016;**15**:671-673. DOI: 10.1586/14760584.2016.1161511

[52] Zlamy M. Rediscovering pertussis. Frontiers in Pediatrics. 2016;**4**:52. DOI: 10.3389/fped.2016.00052

[53] McGuirk P, Heininger U. Protecting newborns from pertussis—The challenge of complete cocooning. BMC Infectious Diseases. 2014;**14**:397. DOI: 10.1186/1471-2334-14-397

[54] Healy CM, Rench MA, Wootton SH, Sastagnini LA. Evaluation of the impact of a pertussis cocooning program on infant pertussis infection. The Pediatric Infectious Disease Journal. 2015;**34**:22-26. DOI: 10.1097/INF.0000000000000486

[55] Frère J, De Wals P, Ovetchkine P, Coïc L, Audibert F, et al. Evaluation of several approaches to immunize parents of neonates against *B. pertussis*. Vaccine. 2013;**31**:6087-6091. DOI: 10.1016/j.vaccine.2013.09.043

[56] De Greeff SC, de Melker HE, Westerhof A, Schellekens JF, Mooi FR, et al. Estimation of household transmission rates of pertussis and the effect of cocooning vaccination strategies on infant pertussis. Epidemiology. 2012;**23**:852-860. DOI: 10.1097/EDE.0b013e31826c2b9e

[57] Marchant A, Sadarangani M, Garand M, Dauby N, Verhasselt V, et al. Maternal immunization: Collaborating with mother nature. The Lancet Infectious Diseases. 2017;**17**:e197-e208

[58] Rivero-Santana A, Cuéllar-Pompa L, Sánchez-Gómez LM, Perestelo-Pérez L, Serrano-Aguilar P. Effectiveness and cost-effectiveness of different immunization strategies against whooping cough to reduce child morbidity and mortality. Health Policy. 2014;**115**:82-91. DOI: 10.1016/j.healthpol.2013.12.007

[59] Tiwari TS, Baughman AL, Clark TA. First pertussis vaccine dose and prevention of infant mortality. Pediatrics. 2015;**135**:990-999. DOI: 10.1542/peds.2014-2291

[60] Abu-Raya B, Srugo I, Kessel A, Peterman M, Bader D, et al. The effect of timing of maternal tetanus, diphtheria, and acellular pertussis (Tdap) immunization during pregnancy on newborn pertussis antibody levels—A prospective study. Vaccine. 2014;**32**:5787-5793. DOI: 10.1016/j.vaccine.2014.08.038

[61] Eberhardt CS, Blanchard-Rohner G, Lemaître B, Boukrid M, Combescure C, et al. Maternal immunization earlier in pregnancy maximizes antibody transfer and expected infant seropositivity against pertussis. Clinical Infectious Diseases. 2016;**62**:829-836. DOI: 10.1093/cid/ciw027

[62] Gall SA, Myers J, Pichichero M. Maternal immunization with tetanus—Diphtheria pertussis vaccine: Effect on maternal and neonatal serum antibody levels. American Journal of Obstetrics and Gynecology. 2011;**204**:e1-e5. DOI: 10.1016/j.ajog.2010.11.024

[63] Hardy-Fairbanks AJ, Pan SJ, Decker MD, Johnson DR, Greenberg DP, et al. Immune responses in infants whose mothers received Tdap vaccine during pregnancy. The Pediatric Infectious Disease Journal. 2013;**32**:1257-1260. DOI: 10.1097/INF.0b013e3182a09b6a

[64] UK Department of Health. Pregnant Women to be Offered Whooping Cough Vaccination. 2015. Available from: http://www.dh.gov.uk/health/2012/09/whooping-cough/ [Accessed: 2017.07.16]

[65] Centers for Disease Control and Prevention. Updated recommendations for use of tetanus toxoid, reduced diphtheria toxoid, and acellular pertussis vaccine (Tdap) in pregnant women—Advisory Committee on Immunization Practices (ACIP), 2012. MMWR. Morbidity and Mortality Weekly Report. 2013;**62**:131-135

[66] Amirthalingam G, Andrews N, Campbell H, Ribeiro S, Kara E, et al. Effectiveness of maternal pertussis vaccination in England: An observational study. Lancet. 2014;**384**:1521-1528. DOI: 10.1016/S0140-6736(14)60686-3

[67] Dabrera G, Amirthalingam G, Andrews N, Campbell H, Ribeiro S, et al. A case-control study to estimate the effectiveness of maternal pertussis vaccination in protecting newborn infants in England and Wales, 2012–2013. Clinical Infectious Diseases. 2015;**60**:333-337. DOI: 10.1093/cid/ciu821

[68] Heininger U. Pertussis: What the pediatric infectious disease specialist should know. The Pediatric Infectious Disease Journal. 2012;**31**:78-79. DOI: 10.1097/INF.0b013e31823b034e

[69] Niewiesk S. Maternal antibodies: Clinical significance, mechanism of interference with immune responses, and possible vaccination strategies. Frontiers in Immunology. 2014;**5**: 446. DOI: 10.3389/fimmu.2014.00446

[70] Eberhardt CS, Blanchard-Rohner G, Lemaître B, Combescure C, Othenin GV, et al. Pertussis antibody transfer to preterm neonates after second-versus third-trimester maternal immunization. Clinical Infectious Diseases. 2017;**64**:1129-1132. DOI: 10.1093/cid/cix046

[71] Ladhani SN, Andrews NJ, Southern J, Jones CE, Amirthalingam G, et al. Antibody responses after primary immunization in infants born to women receiving a pertussis-containing vaccine during pregnancy: Single arm observational study with a historical comparator. Clinical Infectious Diseases. 2015;**61**:1637-1644. DOI: 10.1093/cid/civ695

[72] Melvin JA, Scheller EV, Miller JF, Cotter PA. *Bordetella pertussis* pathogenesis: Current and future challenges. Nature Reviews. Microbiology. 2014;**12**:274-288. DOI: 10.1038/nrmicro3235

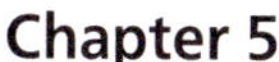

Chapter 5

Pertussis Immunization in Pregnancy: A Review

Giovanni Gabutti, Armando Stefanati and Parvanè Kuhdari

Additional information is available at the end of the chapter

http://dx.doi.org/10.5772/intechopen.72085

Abstract

The pregnant woman has an altered immune response and, for some pathologies, is at increased risk of infection and of developing complications and serious outcomes. In addition, maternal infections can result in congenital anomalies, malformations or severe neonatal diseases. Vaccination of pregnant women can therefore have a double goal: to protect the mother from diseases that could have an impact on her health and to avoid infection/disease transmission to the fetus or the newborn. Despite the potential benefits of immunization in pregnant women, it is still evident reluctance and/or refusal of vaccinations by health professionals as well as by pregnant women, who are wary of the real advantages linked to vaccines. Concerning pertussis, immunization is strongly recommended in pregnancy and some data are already available in Europe as well as in other parts of the world. This review describes the rationale for this immunization and summarizes available data around the world.

Keywords: pertussis, whooping cough, maternal immunization, pregnancy

1. Introduction

Pertussis (or whooping cough) is a worldwide endemic-epidemic respiratory infection, caused by *Bordetella pertussis*, a Gram-negative, aerobic, capsulated bacillus.

Since the 1950s, first, the development of whole-cell and subsequently of acellular vaccines, which may be administered in combination with other antigens (e.g., diphtheria and tetanus toxoids), had a huge impact on the incidence of pertussis and on infant mortality, regardless of the type of vaccine and of the immunization schedule used. However, the duration of protection is not long-lasting, but ranges between 4 and 20 years after natural infection and 4 and 12 years after vaccination [1]. This involved, in particular in the presence of high vaccine coverage, a shift

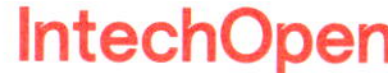

of infection to older age groups, with often unspecific and unrecognized clinical features. Adult subjects with atypical pertussis, often asymptomatic or paucisymptomatic, can become a source of infection for younger children, especially those younger than 2 months of age, who have not yet started the vaccination programs for infants [2] .

A possible solution to limit the likelihood that an infant can be infected during the first months of life is mother's immunization during pregnancy.

Two important results could be achieved through this approach: the first is placental transmission of immunity induced by vaccination; the second is to prevent the mother from being a potential source of infection for the infant.

In the light of the positive experiences of some countries that have recently introduced vaccination in pregnancy, such as USA, Canada, Australia, and UK, vaccination in the third trimester of pregnancy appears to be one of the cornerstones for the prevention of this infection in infants [3].

2. Etiopathogenic and immunological aspects

The transmission of *B. pertussis*, which is an exclusively human and airborne pathogen, occurs through Flügge droplets. The pathogen is characterized by a high basic reproduction number (R0), and for this, it is highly contagious. The infection predominantly affects children and still represents one of the most important causes of death in subjects younger than 1 year of age [4].

Once introduced into the respiratory tract, the pathogen adheres to the ciliary cells of the epithelium by means of adhesins (FHA: filamentous hemagglutinin, FIM1, 2 and 3: fimbriae, PRN: pertactin) and exerts its pathogenic action through the production of some toxins (PT: pertussis toxin PT, AC: adenylated cyclase, DNT: dermonecrotic toxin, TCT: cytotoxin). Adhesins and toxins (TCT excluded) are highly immunogenic [5].

During the incubation period, *B. pertussis* replication, colonization of the respiratory tract, and production of large amounts of toxins occur, causing damage to the epithelium. The toxicity caused by *B. pertussis* stimulates the production of proinflammatory cytokines (IL-1, INF-α, and IL-6) in host cells, responsible for the clinical picture together with the nitric oxide production [5].

Published data show that *B. pertussis* strains evolved over time, with different isolates in pre- and post-immunization ages. Changes in genomic sequences of virulence factors such as PT, FIM, and PRN have been observed in circulating strains. So far, there is no evidence that the effectiveness of whole-cell vaccines decreases due to a continued selection of less susceptible clones to vaccines [6]. In regions where acellular vaccines are in use, the circulation of PRN-negative bacteria, in which the antigen contained in the vaccine is unexpressed, has recently been detected [7]. Very recently, a strain which does not express either PRN or PT has also been described [8].

However, no significant changes in the efficacy of acellular vaccines have been documented, despite the spreading of these new variants of *B. pertussis* [7, 9].

3. Epidemiology

Before the availability of the pertussis vaccine (introduced in the 1950s), about 80% of cases occurred in children <5 years and less than 3% of cases in subjects ≥15 years of age [2].

In 1974, vaccination was included in the "Expanded Programme on immunization" by World Health Organization (WHO), which allowed a gradual increase in vaccine coverage (CV); in 2008, 82% of newborns had received three doses of pertussis vaccine (avoiding 687,000 deaths) and in 2014, the CV was estimated almost equal to 86% [2, 3].

Despite the excellent results related to the worldwide extensive vaccination, WHO data estimated 16 million cases of pertussis in 2010 (95% of which in developing countries), and 195,000 deaths in the pediatric population. In 2013, pertussis caused about 63,000 deaths in children under the age of 5 years [10].

In the USA, the latest CDC estimates reported 15,737 cases in 2016, with a 86% vaccine coverage with three doses. In particular, an incidence rate of 85.5/100,000 and a percentage of hospitalizations of 44% has been registered in children <6 months of age. In children between 6 and 11 months, incidence rate was 27.1/100,000, and 11.9% of them were hospitalized. In the same year, 7 deaths were registered; 6 of them involved <1 year old subjects [11].

With the introduction of vaccination programs, pertussis spreading has shifted to older age groups, thus involving adolescents and adults.

Accordingly to WHO data, this shift may be related to several factors, such as the increased recognition of less frequent manifestations of pathology in older adults, the use of more sensitive lab tests, a more accurate surveillance system that covers the entire life span, and the progressive decay of protective immunity related to a reduction in natural boosters [2].

However, the highest rates of morbidity and mortality attributable to pertussis are reported in children <1 year of age, especially in infants younger than 2 months of age [12]. Infants usually start immunization generally not before 2 months of age and this involves a time frame during which the risk of acquiring pertussis infection transmitted by family members and caregivers (mother, older siblings, grandparents, etc.) is very high [13].

4. Clinical aspects

Clinical presentation is strictly related to the age of acquisition of the infection, the level of immunity, and the use of antibiotic therapy [14].

The disease affects all age groups, especially children, and is one of the most important causes of deaths of <1 year old infants.

The severity of clinical manifestations is inversely related to the age of affected subjects. In children who have not yet been vaccinated, pertussis has a typical course and can lead to major symptoms with severe complications [15]. The prognosis between the first and second year of life is particularly severe, with a high incidence as well as a high number of hospital admissions and deaths (0.2% and 4% lethality rates in developed and developing countries, respectively) [16].

The pertussis incubation period generally lasts 7–10 days, with a range between 4 and 21 days; rarely, it can last up to 42 days. The typical course of the disease is divided into three phases. The first one, called "catarrhal stage," is characterized by the onset of rhinitis, sneezing, fever, and occasional mild coughing. The cough gradually becomes stiffer, and after 1–2 weeks, the second phase, called "paroxysmal stage" begins. Fever is generally low throughout the duration of the disease. It is during the paroxysmal stage that the diagnosis of pertussis can be suspected. Coughing is typical, generally violent, with sudden and paroxysmal attacks, frequently followed by vomiting. It is generally an expression of the difficulty of ejecting the mucus from the tracheobronchial tract. At the end of the paroxysmal attack, a long high-pitched whoop sound or gasp occurs (except in newborns) [17].

Paroxysmal episodes are often followed by physical prostration. In the period between an episode and the other, the subject does not look ill. Paroxysmal attacks occur more frequently at night, with an average of 15 attacks in 24 hours. During the first 1 or 2 weeks of the paroxysmal phase, the attacks increase in frequency, remain stable for another 2–3 weeks and then gradually decrease. The paroxysmal stage usually lasts from 1 to 6 weeks, but can persist up to 10 weeks. In the third phase, "convalescence stage," there is a gradual recovery; paroxysmal cough attacks are less common and tend to disappear in 2 or 3 weeks. However, paroxysmal attacks can occur again, for many months after the onset of pertussis, in the case of concomitant respiratory infections.

The abovementioned description refers to pertussis in its typical form and without therapeutic intervention. Antibiotics significantly improve the clinical picture. The classic presentation of pertussis occurs less frequently even after vaccination [18].

Adolescents, adults, and partially immunized children may have a milder course of disease than babies and infants; the infection can be asymptomatic or can present with symptoms ranging from mild cough to a classical pertussis with persistent cough. Although the disease may be milder in elderly people, such subjects may transmit the infection to other susceptible subjects, including unimmunized or not completely vaccinated infants [19].

The most common complication and cause of death related to pertussis is secondary bacterial pneumonia (about 10% of cases). Neurological complications, such as seizures and encephalopathy, are more common among newborns and may occur as a result of hypoxia or toxin-induced damage. Other less severe complications include otitis media, anorexia, and dehydration. Complications due to paroxysmal attacks include pneumothorax, epistaxis, conjunctival hemorrhage, subdural hematomas, hernias, and rectal prolapse [17, 20].

5. Immunological aspects

After natural infection, anti-PT antibodies (the only *B. pertussis* specific antigen) are found in 80–85% of patients [2]. Antibodies to different *B. pertussis* antigens are believed to play a key role in protecting from the disease (as they neutralize bacterial toxins, inhibit the bond between the bacterium and the respiratory tract cells, and allow the capture and destruction of the bacterium by macrophages and neutrophils). Nevertheless, any specific antibody level, against a single antigen or a combination of antigens, which can be related to clinical protection, is currently unknown [21].

Immunity, whether natural or acquired by vaccination, is not long-lasting and tends to decline in a 4–12 years time range. This data is confirmed by the occurrence of epidemics especially in adolescents and adults, even in geographical areas where vaccine coverage is high. Reinfections may occur in adolescents and adults and have been reported in children as well. It is also well known that cell-mediated immunity plays a key role in protecting against infection; the development of this response can be very important in the clearance of the microorganism and in the subsequent protection [22, 23].

Although there is a placental transmission of maternal antibodies, most newborns do not appear to be protected against the disease during the first months of life, probably due to the low and inadequate levels of antibody transferred, unless the mother has been recently vaccinated. Several studies on maternal immunization have evaluated its validity, demonstrating an effective antibody-mediated protection of infants [24].

6. Available vaccines

The WHO, in the "position paper" on pertussis vaccination published in 2015 [2], points out that the primary goal of immunization should be to reduce the risk of severe forms in childhood, when morbidity and mortality are particularly high, and indicates 90% as the minimum level of coverage to be achieved with three doses in infants, starting vaccination at 6 weeks of age.

Historically, vaccination is carried out using two types of vaccine: whole or old generation vaccine and acellular or new generation vaccine. Both are mainly used as components of combined products (along with diphtheria and tetanus toxoid) in a 3-dose vaccine schedule.

The whole cell vaccine, consisting of inactivated bacteria, showed a highly variable efficacy (36–96%) and a relatively high reactogenicity in several clinical trials, and for this reason, its wide-scale use was limited [25–27]. The use of the whole cell vaccine may correlate with relatively frequent adverse reactions (AE) (26–40% of doses) such as fever, irritability, reactions at the inoculation site, or more rare AE, such as hypotonia-hyporesponsiveness (1/1500–2000 doses) [28, 29]. The proportion of local reactions tends to increase with the increase of age and of the number of administered doses; for these reasons, whole cell vaccines are not recommended in adolescents and adults [29].

Acellular vaccines are less reactogenic [30] and, thanks to their better safety and tolerability profile, their introduction has led to a gradual increase in coverage rates in most Western countries and, consequently, to a significant reduction in the incidence of the disease.

However, several studies have shown that the effectiveness of acellular vaccines decreases over time, leading to an increase in pertussis incidence after 8–12 years, even in areas with high vaccine coverage; this disadvantage has been reduced but not eliminated by using booster doses of reduced antigenic vaccine (ap) [31–33]. The duration of protection, however, tends to decrease, regardless of the administration of whole or acellular vaccine [34].

The introduction of pertussis vaccines, especially acellular ones, has certainly resulted in a strong containment of the incidence of disease, as a result of a gradual increase in vaccine coverage in most Western countries.

However, the illusion of having found a suitable tool to solve a relevant public health problem such as pertussis was short-lived. Since the early 2000s, a rise in pertussis incidence has been observed in several geographic areas, even where high vaccine coverage has been achieved for a long time [35]. This scenario underlines the need to identify a vaccine strategy that prevents the circulation of infection in all age groups and that, above all, helps to prevent illness in infants who have the highest risk of severe and even deadly complications.

7. Cocoon strategy

For several years, the cocoon strategy, which foresees the protection of infants in the first months of life through vaccination of the mother in postpartum and of the family contacts as potential sources of infection, has been considered a promising strategy of vaccination [2].

The rationale of this approach is related to fact that the source of infection for the newborn is represented by parents (5–55% of cases), grandparents (6–8%), and siblings (up to 20%) [36, 37].

However, it is necessary to consider that the maximum immunological response to vaccination does not occur within 14 days after the administration of a booster dose and, for this reason, postpartum immunization does not allow to immediately protect the mother [38].

Anyway, the cocooning was recommended in the early 2000s in some developed countries and since 2005 by ACIP [39, 40].

This strategy has not been completely successful for several reasons [41]: the poor effectiveness, due to the large number of subjects to be vaccinated in order to prevent a single case of pertussis; the inadequate acceptance by family and close contacts of the newborn, especially if there is no pertussis epidemic ongoing (which leads to a perceived low risk); the difficulty in reaching all potential candidates for vaccination, especially if large families are involved; the high economic resources needed to implement such a program in all newborns.

A study conducted in Italy has calculated the number needed to vaccinate (NNV) within the cocoon strategy, that is, the number of people to be vaccinated in order to prevent one hospitalization due to pertussis in 1 year in children <12 months old. The NNV was very high, ranging between 5404 and 9289, depending on the considered variables [42].

The difficulties in implementing the cocoon strategy, its related high costs, and the not completely satisfactory results achieved, lead to the design of a new approach, which is currently considered the main strategy: woman's vaccination during pregnancy.

8. Immunization in pregnancy

Vaccination of pregnant women with dTpa vaccine is nowadays considered the best strategy for the protection of <2 months of age infants, which are a high-risk cohort being too young to be vaccinated.

However, vaccination during pregnancy has been considered for a long time a negligible option because of the difficulty to assess its effectiveness and safety.

The rationale for vaccination in pregnancy with a single dose of dTap is to provide protection against pertussis to the baby in his first months of life through the transplacental passage of maternal antibodies. One of the concerns firstly considered was the possible interference of maternal antibodies on the child's ability to mount an adequate immune response to pediatric DTaP or to other conjugated vaccines containing tetanus or diphtheria toxoids. Other concerns were related to the lack of data on safety and potential teratogenicity. However, now it is well known that there are no potentially serious adverse events in either the mother or the fetus following vaccination during pregnancy [43, 44]. One of the issues for the development of recommendations addressed to immunization of women during pregnancy and lactation is the lack of studies to make evidence-based decisions. Most of the available data on vaccine safety are derived from passive surveillance records. According to the CDC, the risk of a fetus following mother's vaccination during pregnancy is only theoretical. However, when considering vaccination, it is important to distinguish between live and inactivated vaccines. In particular, there is no theoretical reason to suspect that inactivated, bacterial or toxoid vaccines (pertussis one included), are associated with an increased risk of adverse events when given during pregnancy or lactation [45].

As of 2008 [46], the Advisory Committee on Immunization Practices (ACIP) recommended that pregnant women not previously vaccinated with dTap should receive a dose in the immediate postpartum period prior to hospital discharge; could receive dTap even a 2-year interval after a previous dose of dT vaccine; should receive dT during pregnancy as protection against tetanus and diphtheria when indicated; could postpone dT vaccine during pregnancy and replace it with dTap vaccine in the immediate postpartum period, if sufficient protection against tetanus and diphtheria was already available. In conclusion, although there were no contraindications for the administration of dTap vaccine during pregnancy, healthcare professionals had to evaluate risks and benefits before deciding to administer dTap to a pregnant woman.

Subsequently, an analysis was performed comparing immunization in pregnancy to postpartum vaccination in terms of impact, effectiveness, and costs [47]. Vaccination during pregnancy turned out to allow to prevent more cases of disease, hospitalization, and death than the postpartum approach for two reasons: first, because protection is achieved for both the mother and the child at birth; second, because vaccination, when performed during the third trimester of gestation, optimizes the transplacental transfer of maternal antibodies to the fetus, ensuring protection for the newborn during his first months of life.

Based on this evidence, ACIP [48] recommended in 2011 the use of dTpa to all pregnant women who had not previously received the vaccine. The vaccine has to be administered between the end of the second and the beginning of the third trimester, preferably after the 20th week. If the vaccine has not been given during pregnancy, one dose of dTap should be given immediately after delivery. In 2012, the recommendation was extended to all women at each new pregnancy, regardless of their previous vaccination status [48].

This indication was based on the results of some studies which showed that the production of protective antibodies after vaccination is maximum in the first month and is much lower even after less than 1 year; after 1 year, the antibody protection provided by the mother is no longer sufficient to protect the baby in his first months of life, unless vaccination is made during pregnancy. It has been confirmed that dTap administration should preferably take place during the second trimester of gestation, especially between the 27th and 36th week [49, 50], although a study conducted by Abu Raya et al. has shown that avidity of IgG antibodies against *Bordetella pertussis* is greater if vaccination is performed between the 27th and 30th week of gestation [51, 52].

Recently, an observational perspective study [53] has been conducted in Switzerland to evaluate the best time for maternal vaccination in order to adequately protect preterm infants who, among newborns, are a group even more susceptible and at risk. Antibody levels, expressed as geometric mean titers, were evaluated in preterm children born from two cohorts of women vaccinated with dTap, one in the second and one in the third trimester. The results showed a significantly higher level of antibodies in infants born from mothers vaccinated in the second compared to those vaccinated in the third trimester. One possible explanation is that immunization during the second trimester allows a longer transfer time and a higher accumulation of antibodies in newborns This is the first study showing the benefits of maternal immunization in the second trimester for preterm infants. Noteworthy, these interesting results have to be validated as it is well known that the placental transfer of antibodies is greatly effective during the last trimester of pregnancy.

There is no evidence of adverse effects on the fetus after maternal vaccination with inactivated or toxoid vaccines, and coadministration of dTap and flu vaccines is allowed, and it is safe in pregnancy and can optimize the immune response [54, 55].

A study conducted in New Zealand evaluated the safety of dTap vaccine administered during pregnancy; a cohort of 403 newborns was followed for 6–12 months after birth (84% of whom completed a 12-months follow-up), monitoring over time the onset of possible adverse effects related to vaccination. Several parameters such as gestational age at birth, growth parameters, evidence of congenital abnormalities, immunization status, timeliness of immunization, and possible appearance of pertussis infection after birth were considered. The study showed that there were no significant differences in birth weight, gestational age at birth, congenital anomalies or altered growth parameters, comparing newborns from immunized or unvaccinated mothers. No cases of pertussis occurred in the cohort studied, in spite of the high rates of disease in the community and there were no adverse events related to vaccination. Therefore, these data can be added to the growing pool of evidence that dTap vaccine administration during pregnancy is an adequate and safe strategy to reduce the impact of pertussis in infants [56].

In the United States, the CDC recommends a dose of dTap at each pregnancy, between the 27th and 36th week of gestation (preferably between 28th and 32th). dTap vaccine is also recommended in the immediate postpartum, before discharge from the hospital, for mothers who have not received dTap in pregnancy or for those with an unknown vaccination status [48].

In Canada, the National Advisory Committee on Immunization (NACI) recommends that all women who have not received a dose of dTpa vaccine after 26 weeks of pregnancy should be encouraged to undergo vaccination. In particular circumstances, such as in an epidemic situation, all women over the 26th gestation week may be offered dTap regardless of their previous immunological condition [57].

Since 2013, in New Zealand, vaccination is recommended for every new pregnancy between the 28th and 38th week of gestation [58]. In Australia, the guidelines in the latest edition of "The Australian Immunization Handbook" recommend a booster dose for all women in the third trimester of each pregnancy (preferably between the 28th and the 32nd week) [59].

In Europe, following the 2012 epidemic, the United Kingdom launched an immunization program for pregnant women offering vaccination between the 16th and 32nd week of gestation [60]. Belgium (week 24–32), Ireland (week 27–36), Czech Republic (week 28–36) [61], and Italy (after the 28th week) [62] recommend vaccination in pregnancy.

9. Conclusions

Although the impact of pertussis has been considerably reduced since the introduction of vaccination programs in the 1950s, the disease continues to be a public health issue, especially in children in their first months of life.

The spread of *B. pertussis* in the cohort of infants is facilitated by the circulation of the pathogen among older age groups (where cases are often atypical and misdiagnosed) that easily become sources of infection for unvaccinated children. The shift of the disease to the older age groups is related to waning immunity occurring after both natural infection and immunization.

It is therefore necessary to implement vaccination strategies taking into account the most vulnerable groups. On one hand, it is recommended to administer booster doses with dTpa vaccine every 10 years to maintain effective immune protection in previously vaccinated population. On the other hand, it is necessary to adopt a preventive strategy addressed to younger babies, already starting immunization in the prenatal age. Women's vaccination in the third trimester of pregnancy appears to be an effective tool as it allows, through the transplacental passage of specific antibodies, newborn's protection in the first few months of life, at least until he reaches the right age to start immunization.

For a more complete protection of the infant, it would be desirable to simultaneously promote the cocoon strategy, immunizing all members of the family and those who will be in close contact with the newborn, to avoid the transmission of the bacterium by these subjects.

Given the new epidemiological situation and on the basis of the scientific evidence, vaccination in the third trimester of pregnancy is currently recommended in several countries such as the United States, Canada, Australia and other European countries (UK, Italy, etc.).

Conflict of interest

Gabutti G received grants from GlaxoSmithKline Biologicals SA, Sanofi Pasteur MSD, Novartis, Crucell/Janssen, Sequirus, Pfizer MSD Italy and Sanofi Pasteur for being consultant or taking part in advisory boards, expert meetings, being a speaker or an organizer of congresses/conferences, and acting as investigator in clinical trials. Gabutti G has no competing interest related to the content of this article. The other authors have no competing interest.

Author details

Giovanni Gabutti[1]*, Armando Stefanati[1] and Parvanè Kuhdari[2]

*Address all correspondence to: giovanni.gabutti@unife.it

1 Department of Medical Sciences, University of Ferrara, Ferrara, Italy

2 Post-graduate School of Hygiene and Preventive Medicine, University of Ferrara, Ferrara, Italy

References

[1] Wendelboe AM, Van Rie A, Salmaso S, Englund JA. Duration of immunity against pertussis after natural infection or vaccination. The Pediatric Infectious Disease Journal. 2005;**24**(5 Suppl):S58-S61

[2] World Health Organization (WHO). Pertussis vaccines: WHO position paper, August 2015-recommendations. Vaccine. 2016;**34**(12):1423-1425. DOI: 10.1016/j.vaccine.2015.10.136

[3] Gabutti G, Tozzi AE, Bonanni P, Azzari C, Ercolani M, Fuiano L, Prato R, Zuccotti G, Zanetti A. Epidemiologia, vaccinazione e strategie di prevenzione della pertosse in Italia. Rivista Immunologia Allergologia Pediatrica. 2014;**2**(3 Suppl):1-22

[4] Kretzschmar M, Teunis PFM, Pebody RG. Incidence and reproductive numbers of pertussis: estimates form serological and social contact data in five European countries. PLoS Medicine. 2010;**7**:e1000291

[5] Fedele A, Bianco M, Ausiello CM. The virulence factors of Bordetella pertussis: Talented modulators of host immune response. Archivum Immunologiae et Therapiae Experimentalis. 2013;**61**:445-457

[6] Hegerle N, Guiso N. Epidemiology of whooping cough & typing of Bordetella pertussis. Future Microbiology. 2013;**8**(11):1391-1403. DOI: 10.2217/fmb.13.111

[7] Hegerle N, Guiso N. Bordetella pertussis and pertactin-deficient clinical isolates: Lessons for pertussis vaccines. Expert Review of Vaccines. 2014;**13**(9):1135-1146. DOI: 10.1586/14760584.2014.932254

[8] Williams MM, Sen K, Weigand MR, Skoff TH, Cunningham VA, Halse TA, Tondella ML, CDC Pertussis Working Group. Bordetella pertussis strain lacking pertactin and pertussis toxin. Emerging Infectious Diseases 2016;**22**(2):319-322. Doi:10.3201/eid2202.151332

[9] Mooi FR, He Q, Guiso N. Phylogeny, evolution and epidemiology of Bordetellae. In: Locht C, editor. Bordetella: Molecular Microbiology. 1st ed. Norfolk, UK: Horizon Bioscience; 2007. pp. 17-45

[10] World Health Organization (WHO). Global Health Observatory Data Repository. [Internet]. Available from: http://apps.who.int/gho/data/node.main.ChildMortREG100?lang=en. [Accessed: Oct 10, 2017]

[11] Center for Disease Control and Prevention (CDC). Provisional Pertussis Surveillance Report. [Internet]. 2016. Available from: https://www.cdc.gov/pertussis/downloads/pertuss-surv-report-2016-provisional.pdf. [Accessed: Oct 10, 2017]

[12] Robinson CL, Romero JR, Kempe A, Pellegrini C. Advisory committee on immunization practices recommended immunization schedule for children and adolescents aged 18 years or younger. United States 2017. MMWR – Morbidity and Mortality Weekly Report. 2017;**66**:134-135. DOI: http://dx.doi.org/10.15585/mmwr.mm6605e1

[13] Skoff TH, Kenyon C, Cocoros N, Liko J, Miller L, Kudish K, Baumbach J, Zansky S, Faulkner A, Martin SW. Sources of infant pertussis infection in the United States. Pediatrics. 2015;**136**(4):635-641. DOI: 10.1542/peds.2015-1120

[14] Heininger U, Stehr K, Cherry JD. Serious pertussis overlooked in infants. European Journal of Pediatrics. 1992;**151**:342-343

[15] Gabutti G, Rota MC. Pertussis: A review of disease epidemiology worldwide and in Italy. International Journal of Environmental Research and Public Health. 2012;**9**(12):4626-4638

[16] Blangiardi F, Ferrera G. Reducing the risk of pertussis in newborn infants. Journal of Preventive Medicine and Hygiene. 2009;**50**(4):206-216

[17] Center for Disease Control and Prevention (CDC). Pertussis. [Internet]. Available from: https://www.cdc.gov/vaccines/pubs/pinkbook/pert.html. [Accessed: Oct 10, 2017]

[18] Cherry JD, Grimprel E, Guiso N, Heininger U, Mertsola J. Defining pertussis epidemiology: Clinical, microbiologic and serologic perspectives. The Pediatric Infectious Disease Journal. 2005;**24**(5 Suppl):S25-S34

[19] Spector TB, Maziarz EK. Pertussis. The Medical Clinics of North America. 2013;**97**(4):537-552, ix. DOI: 10.1016/j.mcna.2013.02.004

[20] Greenberg DP, Von Konig CH, Heininger U. Health burden of pertussis in infants and children. The Pediatric Infectious Disease Journal. 2005;**24**(S5):39-43

[21] Higgs R, Higgins SC, Ross PJ, Mills KH. Immunity to the respiratory pathogen Bordetella pertussis. Mucosal Immunology. 2012;**5**(5):485-500. DOI: 10.1038/mi.2012.54

[22] Edelman K, He Q, Mäkinen J, Sahlberg A, Haanperä M, Schuerman L, Wolter J, Mertsola J. Immunity to pertussis 5 years after booster immunization during adolescence. Clinical Infectious Diseases. 2007;**44**(10):1271-1277

[23] World Health Organization (WHO). Module 4: pertussis-update 2009. In: Department of Immunization, Vaccines and Biologicals, editor. The Immunological Basis for Immunization Series. Geneva: World Health Organization. 2010;1-37. Available from: http://apps.who.int/iris/handle/10665/44311. [Accessed: 10-10-2017]

[24] Amirthalingam G, Andrews N, Campbell H, Ribeiro S, Kara E, Donegan K, Fry NK, Miller E, Ramsay M. Effectiveness of maternal pertussis vaccination in England: An observational study. Lancet. 2014;**384**(9953):1521-1528. DOI: 10.1016/S0140-6736(14)60686-3

[25] Cherry JD. Historical review of pertussis and the classical vaccine. The Journal of Infectious Diseases. 1996;**174**(3 Suppl):S259-S263

[26] Mooi FR, van Loo IHM, King AJ. Adaptation of Bordetella pertussis to vaccination: A cause for its reemergence? Emerging Infectious Diseases 2001;**7**:526-528

[27] Dias WO, van der Ark AA, Sakauchi MA, Kubrusly FS, Prestes AF, Borges MM, Furuyama N, Horton DS, Quintilio W, Antoniazi M, Kuipers B, van der Zeijst BA, Raw I. An improved whole cell pertussis vaccine with reduced content of endotoxin. Human Vaccines & Immunotherapeutics 2013;**9**(2):339-348

[28] Bar-On ES, Goldberg E, Hellmann S, Leibovici L. Combined DTPHBV-HIB vaccine versus separately administered DTP-HBV and HIB vaccines for primary prevention of diphtheria, tetanus, pertussis, hepatitis B and haemophilus influenzae b (HIB). Cochrane Database of Systematic Reviews. 2012;**4**:CD005530

[29] World Health Organization (WHO). Pertussis vaccines: WHO position paper. Wkly Epidemiol Rec. 2010;**85**:385-400

[30] Bernstein HH, Rothstein EP, Pichichero ME, Green JL, Reisinger KS, Blatter MM, Halpern J, Arbeter AM, Bernstein DI, Smith V, et al. Reactogenicity and immunogenicity of a three-component acellular pertussis vaccine administered as the primary series to 2, 4 and 6 month old infants in the United States. Vaccine. 1995;**13**:1631-1635

[31] Misegades LK, Winter K, Harriman K, Talarico J, Messonnier NE, Clark TA, Martin SW. Association of childhood pertussis with receipt of 5 doses of pertussis vaccine by time since last vaccine dose, Calfornia, 2010. Journal of the American Medical Association. 2012;**308**:2126-2132

[32] Witt MA, Katz PH, Witt DJ. Unexpectedly limited durability of immunity following acellular pertussis vaccination in preadolescents in a north American outbreak. Clinical Infectious Diseases. 2012;**54**:1730-1735

[33] Witt MA, Arias L, Katz PH, Truong ET, Witt DJ. Reduced risk of pertussis among persons ever vaccinated with whole cell pertussis vaccine compared to recipients of acellular pertussis vaccines in a large US cohort. Clinical Infectious Diseases. 2013;**56**:1248-1254

[34] Zhang L, Prietsch SO, Axelsson I, Halperin SA. Acellular vaccines for preventing whooping cough in children. Cochrane Database of Systematic Reviews. 2012;**3**:CD001478. DOI: 10.1002/14651858

[35] World Health Organization (WHO). Pertussis. [Internet]. Available from: http://www.who.int/immunization/monitoring_surveillance/burden/vpd/surveillance_type/passive/pertussis/en/. [Accessed: 10-10-2017]

[36] Wendelboe AM, Njamkepo E, Bourillon A, Floret DD, Gaudelus J, Gerber M, Grimprel E, Greenberg D, Halperin S, Liese J, Muñoz-Rivas F, Teyssou R, Guiso N, Van Rie A; Infant Pertussis Study Group.Transmission of *Bordetella pertussis* to young infants. The Pediatric Infectious Disease Journal 2007;**26**(4):293-299

[37] Bisgard KM, Pascual FB, Ehresmann KR, Miller CA, Cianfrini C, Jennings CE, Rebmann CA, Gabel J, Schauer SL, Lett SM. Infant pertussis: Who was the source? The Pediatric Infectious Disease Journal. 2004;**23**(11):985-989

[38] Halperin BA, Morris A, Mackinnon-Cameron D, Mutch J, Langley JM, McNeil SA, Macdougall D, Halperin SA. Kinetics of antibody response to tetanus-diphtheria-acellular pertussis vaccine in women with childbearing age and postpartum women. Clinical Infectious Diseases. 2011;**53**:885-892

[39] McIntyre P, Wood N. Pertussis in early infancy: Disease burden and preventive strategies. Current Opinion in Infectious Diseases. 2009;**22**(3):215-223

[40] De La Rocque F, Grimprel E, Gaudelus J, Lécuyer A, Wollner C, Leroux MC, Cohen R. Vaccination in parents of young infants survey. Archives de Pédiatrie. 2007;**14**(12):1472-1476

[41] Forsyth K, Plotkin S, Tan T, Wirsing von König CH. Strategies to decrease pertussis transmission to infants. Pediatrics 2015;**135**:e1475-e1482. doi: 10.1542/peds.2014-3925

[42] Meregaglia M, Ferrara L, Melegaro A, Demicheli V. Parent "cocoon" immunization to prevent pertussis-related hospitalization in infants: The case of Piemonte in Italy. Vaccine. 2013;**31**:1135-1137

[43] Ray P, Hayward J, Michelson D, Lewis E, Schwalbe J, Black S, Shinefield H, Marcy M, Huff K, Ward J, Mullooly J, Chen R, Davis R, Vaccine Safety Datalink GroupEncephalopathy after whole-cell pertussis or measles vaccination: Lack of evidence for a causal association in a retrospective case-control study. The Pediatric Infectious Disease Journal 2006;**25**(9):768-773

[44] Gabutti G, Azzari C, Bonanni P, Prato R, Tozzi AE, Zanetti A, Zuccotti G. Pertussis. Human Vaccines & Immunotherapeutics. 2015;**11**(1):108-117. DOI: 10.4161/hv.34364

[45] Center for Disease Control and Prevention (CDC). General recommendations on immunization: recommendations of the Advisory Committee on Immunization Practices (ACIP). Morbidity and Mortality Weekly Report. 2011;**60**(2):1-60

[46] Murphy TV, Slade BA, Broder KR, Kretsinger K, Tiwari T, Joyce PM, Iskander JK, Brown K, Moran JS; Advisory Committee on Immunization Practices (ACIP) Centers for Disease Control and Prevention (CDC). Prevention of pertussis, tetanus, and diphtheria among

pregnant and postpartum women and their infants recommendations of the Advisory Committee on Immunization Practices (ACIP). MMWR Recommendations and Reports. 2008;**57**(RR-4):1-51

[47] Center for Disease Control and Prevention (CDC). Updated recommendations for use of tetanus toxoid, reduced diphtheria toxoid and acellular pertussis vaccine (Tdap) in pregnant women and persons who have or anticipate having close contact with an infant aged <12 months—Advisory Committee on Immunization Practices (ACIP), 2011. Morbidity and Mortality Weekly Report. 2011;**60**(41):1424-1426

[48] Centers for Disease Control and Prevention (CDC). Updated recommendations for use of tetanus toxoid, reduced diphtheria toxoid, and acellular pertussis vaccine (Tdap) in pregnant women – Advisory Committee on Immunization Practices (ACIP), 2012. Morbidity and Mortality Weekly Report. 2013;**62**(07):131-135

[49] Eberhardt CS, Blanchard-Rohner G, Lemaître B, Combescure C, Othenin-Girard V, Chilin A, Petre J, Martinez de Tejada B, Siegrist CA. Pertussis antibody transfer to preterm neonates after second- versus third-trimester maternal immunization. Clinical Infectious Diseases 2017;**64**(8):1129-1132

[50] Winter K, Cherry JD, Harriman K. Effectiveness of prenatal tetanus, diphtheria, and acellular pertussis vaccination on pertussis severity in infants. Clinical Infectious Diseases. 2017;**64**(1):9-14

[51] Abu Raya B, Bamberger E, Almog M, Peri R, Srugo I, Kessel A. Immunization of pregnant women against pertussis: The effect of timing on antibody avidity. Vaccine. 2015;**33**(16):1948-1952. DOI: 10.1016/j.vaccine.2015.02.059

[52] Gabutti G, Conforti G, Tomasi A, Kuhdari P, Castiglia P, Prato R, Memmini S, Azzari C, Rosati GV, Bonanni P. Why, when and for what diseases pregnant and new mothers "should" be vaccinated. Human Vaccines & Immunotherapeutics. 2017;**13**(2):283-290. DOI: 10.1080/21645515.2017.1264773

[53] Eberhardt CS, Blanchard-Rohner G, Lemaître B, Combescure C, Othenin-Girard V, Chilin A, Petre J, Martinez de Tejada B, Siegrist CA. Pertussis antibody transfer to preterm neonates after second- versus third-trimester maternal immunization. Clinical Infectious Diseases 2017;**64**(8):1129-1132. doi: 10.1093/cid/cix046

[54] McMillan M, Clarke M, Parrella A, Fell DB, Amirthalingam G, Marshall HS. Safety of tetanus, diphtheria, and pertussis vaccination during pregnancy: A systematic review. Obstetrics and Gynecology. 2017;**129**(3):560-573. DOI: 10.1097/AOG.0000000000001888

[55] Sukumaran L, McCarthy NL, Kharbanda EO, Weintraub ES, Vazquez-Benitez G, McNeil MM, Li R, Klein NP, Hambidge SJ, Naleway AL, Lugg MM, Jackson ML, King JP, DeStefano F, Omer SB, Orenstein WA. Safety of tetanus toxoid, reduced diphtheria toxoid, and acellular pertussis and influenza vaccinations in pregnancy. Obstetrics and Gynecology. 2015;**126**(5):1069-1074. DOI: 10.1097/AOG.0000000000001066

[56] Walls T, Graham P, Petousis-Harris H, Hill L, Austin N. Infant outcomes after exposure to Tdap vaccine in pregnancy: An observational study. BMJ Open. 2016;**6**(1):e009536. DOI: 10.1136/bmjopen-2015-009536

[57] Government of Canada. Update on Pertussis Vaccination in Pregnancy. [Internet]. Available from: https://www.canada.ca/en/public-health/services/immunization/national-advisory-committee-on-immunization-naci/update-on-pertussis-vaccination-pregnancy.html. [Accessed: Oct 10, 2017]

[58] The Immunisation Advisory Centre. New Zealand National Immunisation Schedule. [Internet]. Available from: http://www.immune.org.nz/sites/default/files/Immune_Schedule_02-17_4correct%20order.pdf. [Accessed: Oct 10, 2017]

[59] Australian Government. The Australian Immunisation Handbook. 10th ed. 2015. [Internet]. Available from: http://www.immunise.health.gov.au/internet/immunise/publishing.nsf/Content/7B28E87511E08905CA257D4D001DB1F8/$File/Aus-Imm-Handbook.pdf. [Accessed: Oct 10, 2017]

[60] Government of United Kingdom. Vaccination Against Pertussis (Whooping Cough) for Pregnant Women. 2016. [Internet]. Available from: https://www.gov.uk/government/publications/vaccination-against-pertussis-whooping-cough-for-pregnant-women. [Accessed: Oct 10, 2017]

[61] European Centre for Disease Control (ECDC). Vaccination Schedule. [Internet]. Available from: http://vaccine-schedule.ecdc.europa.eu/Pages/Scheduler.aspx. [Accessed: Oct 10, 2017]

[62] Ministero della Salute. Piano Nazionale Prevenzione Vaccinale (PNPV) 2017-2019. [Internet]. Available from: http://www.salute.gov.it/imgs/C_17_pubblicazioni_2571_allegato.pdf. [Accessed: Oct 10, 2017]